BODY BALANCE JUICE PROGRAMME

Body Balance Juice Programme

CLEANSE AND DETOX

Copyright © 2018 by Author Dr. Janet Blair.

For information about special discount for bulk purchases, please contact Thomas Publishing at info@healthscreening vitality.com

First Edition: 2018

ISBN: 978-0-9927743-2-5

www.healthscreeningvitality.com

BODY BALANCE JUICE PROGRAMME

The Road to Feeling Your Best

DETOX, WEIGHT LOSS, INFUSIONS, NUTRITION

Foreword

In 2013, the international trading company I had been working in for 2 years closed its UK head office. After this decision, many long-committed and single parent colleagues supporting their families at home such as myself were unexpectedly stripped of their only source of income.

Being left hung out to dry, I was met by a blinding truth. The story of my life had entered a brand new chapter, one filled with both bewilderment and tragedy. Amid this sudden and uncharted territory, came a subtle warning about the importance of a singular thing; HEALTH!

Just days before I lost my job at the trading company, my 76-year-old mother was diagnosed with several internal problems, including; vascular dementia, renal failure and high blood pressure. Ever since the diagnosis, my mother had been rendered interdependent upon me as her personal but part-time carer.

Therefore, instead of subsequently queuing up in the unemployment line with everyone else, I chose to sacrifice my financial well-being in order to provide a more hospitable home for the soul I loved so dearly.

As I spent long hours during the day bathing, dressing and cooking for her all the while receiving her warm compliments, I began to gradually reflect upon my own health. I wondered, what would I look like once I touch her age? How can I change this? These challenges facing her spurred interest in my own possible health issues, and whilst at an appointment with a health practitioner, they soon became a reality.

"Janet, it appears you have a mass", the male practitioner said "...I believe the problem to be very severe."

I can honestly tell you with my then reasonable skepticism of alternative medicine I refused to foresee the serious implications of his stern warnings that day, and I almost paid the ultimate price.

In the next section of this book, you shall know exactly why this constant neglect of professional help would become my 'Achilles heel'.

Following a succession of problems over the next five years such as lethargic episodes, headaches, swollen feet, dizziness, fainting and no longer being able to dine at my favorite Caribbean restaurants, I was entirely devastated when all these difficulties lead to my final diagnosis of bowel cancer.

Therefore, by this culmination and the fact that I fought and won my battle, I feel empowered to remind readers about the importance of health in the following chapters. I hope that by the end of reading this book, you will have learnt from my experience. You should be convinced that one should not ignore their body, I implore you to respond promptly to whatever signs your body tells you and understand using the information given, how to maintain its vitality through the Body Balance Juice Programme.

I am forever grateful that I found a way to reclaim my health after a devastating diagnosis of bowel cancer. It is my desire to help anyone who may be suffering from ill health so I share my journey with you, and some additional pieces of information.

Please consult with your trusted healthcare provider before embarking on the Body Balance Juice Programme.

www.healthscreeningvitality.com.

Acknowledgments

Beyond measure, thank you God for giving me the insight, inspiration and vision to share my knowledge in this book. Based on my experience you have given me the strength to push forward no matter what life has offered.

I would like to thank my two children; Shanice McAnuff and Jermaine McAnuff for your love and support.

I would also like to extend my thank you to Erran Warden for giving me the opportunity to expand my nutritional knowledge in helping others to identify their health challenges by providing a programme to assist with their health.

Thank you Tony Balhazar for your help as a marketing expert to assist with thinking out of the box and identifying the needs of our community. Thank you also to the graphic designer and other online services.

Thanks to my friends; Sonia Poleon, Serah Lister, Anthony Lyken, Naomi Soako, Claudine Reid, Lara Alao and Patrick Reid who believed I have something to share to encourage change and transform people's lives.

About the Author

At the beginning of the New Year, what do most people do? Make resolutions! Some of us that are fixed upon self-body improvement may include goals such as cutting down on carbs or getting fit and healthy.

So Imagine this. It's the turn of the New Year, a fresh January day, the old calendar has been replaced and your resolutions are clearly set out. Similarly, I recall it being the first day of 2013, where amidst the cold morning breeze I was happily driving to my health practitioner for a full body MOT scan. Far from your routine check-up by the local doctor, today's morning drive was a special day for me, one also unfortunately met by the enemy of typical British traffic. Regardless, I was an unstoppable force motivated by the hope that somehow and some way a 5-minute body scan would miraculously reveal all the health issues that possibly had been lying dormant within me and I would have a chance to solve them.

Much earlier before the New Year I reached out to my alternative health practitioner who informed me of a particular scan machine he owned that could show me various internal ingredients lacking for a completely healthy body and also how to prevent future illnesses.

"The scan works by electronic magnetic fields, it scans the cells in the body; heart, brain, blood, minerals etc. and produces a report that informs a client on what is needed to improve their health followed by a 90 minute consultation."

The thought of actually thwarting illnesses first discovered in my mother from trickling down to me and thus allowing me to relay such precious information onto my children had me giddy and glad more than ever for today. However, this journey to a health practitioner would later prove to be closer to the briefing stage of a mission I was not in the least mentally prepared for. At the end of it, I could hope to secure all the vitality of my health. However achieving this would be miles beyond just frivolous efforts such as piling up the fruit and vegetable basket. Moments later the stationary cars started to move again and so, to the scan it was! I rolled up to the health practitioner's driveway at exactly 11.45 am in front of a great white house. He greeted me with a huge smile behind which appeared to be such a cheerful spirit.

"Hello Janet!" he said, "ready for your scan?"

I nodded in agreement. We casually passed through the house where he guided me into a small office-like room, with facilities limited only to a desk, a black laptop, tiny grey wires and a chair for me to sit in. He then went to fetch some water. Finding the unusual absence of medical equipment, a tad amusing, I thought to myself, "is this all?" Then, like a ghost my health practitioner appeared over the corner of my left shoulder.

"Alright Janet!" he said in the same loud but strangely casual tone "shall we begin?"

I smiled with an added pinch of false confidence. Who knew what kind of scan I would undergo or whether the 5-minute body scan would produce real results? I was ushered into the seat and we began the scanning process; first by pressing my left palm down onto a bloated blue and silver coloured mouse. 'After this, he'll send me away with a get-fit-quick scheme to follow and I'll be free of any unwanted afflictions' or so I thought.

That day, time seemed to pass slower than ever. I am no different from the average person over 40 years of age. Luckily, I've had no symptoms of the serious problems that my elderly mother suffered from, like vascular dementia, renal failure and high blood pressure. I'm almost immune to disease it seems.

I kept glancing over at the overhead clock whose hand appeared to me like it was stuck on exactly one-minute pass twelve. The practitioner asked me jokingly whether I had somewhere else to rush off to, I immediately said 'no...', knowing that I'd been preparing for this since last year September "...but how much longer till some results!?" He chuckled, fully aware of my ignorance, now assuring me that this would be the fastest scan I was going to have in my life.

My anxiety had eased down soon after he'd asked me a series of questions about my health and lifestyle which I found slightly distracting from what was really going on. Nevertheless, I answered accordingly and even in the midst of such a relentless interview, I found the time to daydream about what particular groceries I needed to collect from supermarket before the end of the day. Minutes later when I finally decided break away from my thoughts and to look over at my health practitioner's face, I found his once lively demeanour had since tightened into something more stern. Immediately I felt a chill run down my spine. He caught my gaze thankfully and flashed a pleasant grin which reassured me that everything was in fact okay. So I resumed, until suddenly I was woken by the sound of the machine loudly beeping as the scan drew to its completion.

In silence I waited and pondered over the possible results; he told me he'd be just a moment. Sigh. 'here comes the story of how I should stop eating chocolates, red meat, fried food or worse to actually exercise,' I told myself. However, that stern look on his face, which had grown stricter than a few moments before would not leave, something was holding it there, in a clenching grip, making him appear almost like a statue. In an instant, he drew his face quickly away from the computer in shock and I was now becoming very agitated.

"Well..." I asked letting this one-word question chip away at the stone-hard tension. "...what does it say?"

He leaned over to me struggling to bring back his old joyous self, the corner of his mouth was twitching to force his customary grin and said, "Janet... you are walking dead...".

The scan results revealed several areas in my body that needed immediate attention. He suggested a health programme which involved completely revamping my diet and taking vitamins as well as other supplements to assist me with my health challenges. Two months later I made a vital mistake and gave that up. My reason for it you ask? Addiction mingled in with a little pride.

I was under the impression that if it isn't a disease, then why should I worry? These problems will eventually sort themselves out. Hopefully.

I was still trying to keep fit in other ways assuming this approach served to be a suitable remedy. Over the next three years, I had developed a regular Saturday routine of exercise in a local park with my coach Anthony Lyken, a tall and slender ex-combat engineer solider who served for the US Army and can be quite the joker. I remember it was at the end of those harsh Saturday morning exercise classes at 6:30am that I was strangely met by dizziness, nauseous and intense heat. Anthony often joked that I must have a baby on the way. As funny as it was, I had become a bit concerned about it, whilst also blaming the episodes on a squandered breakfast. 'It should go away in due time though' I thought. For a while, these random disturbances remained quiet but eventually` made their roaring return in a way that rattled any confidence I had that everything going on inside my body was just fine and dandy.

It was April 2015, while on a flight to Australia for a "Date with Destiny" conference hosted by Anthony Robbins, I felt overwhelmingly nauseous. I remembered my doctor warned me to buy over the counter travel sickness tablets before boarding anywhere. I followed his advice exactly and then took some a little more than 3 hours before my 24-hour flight half way across the world. Once air-borne, I called one of sunny flight attendance over for a bottle of lemonade but as I began my request, my stomach growled and I could not finish my sentence. I felt a strong pain.

"Ma'am, are you okay?" she asked in a concerned tone to which I responded with a friendly smile to assert an impression that everything was well, even though this couldn't be further from the truth.

"Fine thanks, just feeling a little sick... may I have some lemonade please?" Minutes went by, then an hour and the problem remained. 'What is wrong with me? 'A voice told me, a trip to the restroom may help and I listened. As my friend was fast asleep I got up onto the aisle towards the restroom. It was at this moment, whilst halfway across the aisle, that I noticed my vision slipping away. Objects began to swirl in a hypnotic manner. Passengers' heads blurred and strangely duplicated themselves into threes. Then, quickly it felt like a dark veil was pulled over my eyes and pitch black darkness took over.

Suddenly, I could smell the stench of old carpet. My eyes sluggishly opened to see feet encircling and standing around me. I didn't realize that I was on the floor outside of a toilet until I heard a member of the cabin crew ask me if I was travelling alone or if I was with someone. That someone, my best friend, happened to be dead asleep at the time. I then realised that I hadn't even made it to my destination. I fainted.

Thankfully, once I had regained consciousness, the cabin crew walked with me to the back of the airplane, away from the swelling drama I had unintentionally stirred up and the passengers that were woken from their sleep. My eyes were half closed and fluttering but with my limited sight I saw one of the cabin crew members kneel down on the floor and lean over towards me. Somehow the after effects of fainting made everything I heard melodic, so instead of plain instructions, his gentle words now jelled into a soothing symphony.

"Sweetheart, we want to see if everything is alright, do you mind walking a little for us?"

It only took a few seconds for them to witness all my collected strength collapse and down I fell again, like a bird out of the sky. What worse is once I came to and was now finally within bounds of my seat I started to vomit right in the aisle of the other passengers. How embarrassing!

Eventually the team managed to place me back in my designated seat and supplied me with an oxygen mask for my recovery. 2 hours passed and I felt ok to travel to my final destination. Meanwhile I kept in mind what a truly telling situation this was. A serious warning, I had again purely out of bad habit, decided to shrug off.

Months later I had the opportunity to speak at a women's event one evening in London called 'Gravity Angels'. Tonight, several entrepreneurial people gathered and were given the chance to promote their businesses through short slide-show presentations. One of the speakers was nutritional therapist Erran Warden, who spoke on the topic "How to promote freedom through well-being." It turned out he was offering the same scan that I had taken in 2013. After the event I decided to introduce myself to him and asked him if he could book me in for a scan. He devised a programme, which I started, but yet again, I chose not to complete.

Then in March 2017, while in attendance at the Holiday Inn Caribbean Night for my friend's 50th birthday, it finally hit me. The intensity of feeling nauseous, dizziness and weakness combining in this one moment meant I could not raise another forkful to my mouth, which is, excuse the exaggeration, unruly! I am Jamaican born and bred. The idea that I could not enjoy a single portion of Caribbean food; curry goat, oxtail, rice and peas, prawns, jerk salmon, is frustrating. The weight of distress was indescribable and now my head lolled embarrassingly across the table in front of friends who soon reclined fearfully in their chairs.

The next day, I had grown weary of my fate and decided to contact Erran to get another scan, which revealed that the ongoing problems I had been experiencing at random were to do with my blood. By this time, I was extremely worried for the sake of my health and would do anything to fix it. The report explained my iron and selenium were low. I was deficient in vitamins and amino acids.

I contacted my General Practitioner (GP) who recommended getting a blood test for confirmation at my local hospital. In addition to this, the blood test confirmed the issues; it showed that my haemoglobin (HB) was very low; 4.9 exactly whereas the average level for a woman ranges from 12.0 – 15.5 grams per decilitre. Alerted by the hospital, I was admitted to be transfused with three units of blood.

My GP, also concerned, suggested that they run other tests such as an endoscopy and colonoscopy. All these various serious sounding tests caused me to panic. Was there an issue deeper than I had suspected all this time? All these years I had been neglecting health advice and happily sinking my teeth into bad meat and sugared delicacies with friends and family, for this?

I was swiftly recommended to the oncologist, but left in the dark as to why. The clinical nurse specialist (CNS) then asked me to come in for a so-called 'brief' consultation. Due to other obligations I told her, I could not attend the appointment until the following week. She stressed to me it was very important that I attend. Scared for my life, I went immediately.

Upon my arrival into the room, she first questioned me as to whether I was alone. I told her yes both my children would not be home until later in the evening and were not available at this time. Immediately after this response I noticed a deep sigh of relief heave out from her chest and she sat me down beside her desk. The results were in. I had bowel cancer. The clinical nurse specialist assured me with confidence that all was not lost and referred me to other suitable colleagues within the medical practice for support. Very rapidly, I found myself placed on an urgent list for surgery to remove the tumour, after which they took a few samples to the lab from the mass to see which stage it was at and if it had spread elsewhere.

Following 3 weeks after the operation of endless waiting and prayer, I received a call from the clinical nurse specialist. I had been praying that the results would be negative.

It was a great relief when the test came back completely negative! The cancer was utterly gone, and even so far removed from my DNA that I could cast away any ounce of anxiety that it may be passed on to my children. Thank God!

Shortly after this scare, I finally took the natural health programme seriously and I must say it has helped me out tremendously. I have lost weight, 20 pounds in fact. I feel much more alert throughout the day and have a better relationship with healthier and nutritious food. Surprisingly I have even succeeded in reducing my shopping bill.

For these reasons, I have chosen to share my story with you. I want to help others reclaim their health, just as I have by first following these carefully guided steps.

J. P. McAnuff

Contents

CHAPTER 1

Before We Get Started...

B efore setting out on this course, it is important to first assess your primary drivers, so that you know if you have met your goal at the end. Why do you want to detox? You may be detoxing to lose weight, clear up your skin, boost your immune system, increase your energy or have fewer aches and pains. This is a very personal goal and important to be noted before embarking on any wellness journey.

Pro Tip

Use your Detox Journal to track your progress. Note your weight, feelings, goals, what you eat and anything else that comes up along the way.

Goal Setting & Using Your Detox Journal

A goal without a plan is just a wish!

So let's go about creating a concrete plan for you to reach your goals.

I have done everything possible to make this a straightforward programme for you to follow. However, you also need to make sure to stick to your end of the bargain and follow the plan closely. As well as this, I would like for you to use your *Body Balance Juice Programme* Journal to map out personal plans and goals.

Goal setting is a powerful process for thinking about your ideal future, and for motivating yourself to turn your vision of this future into reality. A healthy and successful life is nothing more than a lot of successful days strung together. It's going to take so many days to reach your goal; every minute of every day must count.

It will be helpful to see each day as a building block to your perfect life. Each block should not be placed down haphazardly. To create the health and life you want, each day should be treated as a work of art, with all of its ups and downs, those building blocks planned out and placed gently on the foundations that you will be building every day.

Firstly, you must define your health goals and decide to stick with the plan to achieve them.

If you go to your *Body Balance Juice Programme Journal* you will find a list of possible drivers that may be your main reasons for taking part in this programme.

I would like for you to go to the goal setting section of your journal and take 5 minutes to outline your "why" you are taking part in this programme.

I want you to eliminate any short-term wishes to go back to old habits and commit to following the programme for the full 21 days. It will most likely seem hard at times, our mind is great at playing tricks on us and trying to "protect us" by persuading us to do the same thing over and over.

So take it one day at a time. Focus on each day as an individual stepping stone to a healthier, happier you.

Each day, follow the recipes and make sure to fill in your journal to allow you a space to focus on the present day. Take it one step at a time, and be strong. I know you can do this!

CHAPTER 2

What is Natural Detoxing?

Everyone is exposed to toxins on a daily basis, some of which are detrimental to our health. A lot of the toxins we consume in our food are harmless in small doses but build up over time. Detoxing is a process whereby we aim to fully eliminate the toxins in our diet (or as much as possible), thus, allowing our body to heal naturally by releasing any toxins from our body.

Everyone is unique and our abilities to detoxify differ from person to person. That is why one person might get ill with cancer when exposed to carcinogens, whilst another person seems may not be be affected at all.

Our body is very versatile and has the ability to heal itself. We have both internal and external systems for detoxification. The internal systems are the stomach, intestines, liver, immune system, kidneys, lymphatic system and lungs. The external system is primarily our skin which is the largest organ for detoxing in our body.

Reasons for Detoxing your Body

Over the past 100 years we have been exposed to more and more man-made toxins. Although we have built-in mechanisms to remove toxins from our bodies, the overwhelming amount of toxins in our environment means that we all need to be aware of the increased effect they have on our health. Knowing this information and detoxing often will take us closer to a life of health and wellness.

Detoxing can allow you to live a more energetic and healthy life. It has the amazing ability to extend your life.

With more than 84,000 man-made chemicals being released into our environment every year, it is no wonder that our bodies can get toxic overload. There are also natural toxins like bacteria, yeast, mould, fungus and parasites. Toxicity also comes from heavy metals, which builds up over time and can harm our health.

In this day and age, man-made chemicals are in almost everything that we touch, even in the air we breathe. There are also naturally occurring chemicals that can be toxic to our health. That is why our bodies have built-in detoxification systems and antioxidant protection. These systems in our bodies are greatly boosted by maintaining a diet that is rich in fruits and vegetables (especially raw fruit and vegetables).

We are constantly exposed to pesticides and herbicides; these are some of the most damaging to our health. It is important to do a cleanse, every once in a while to help your body flush out excess toxins. Many people opt to cleanse with the seasons; four times a year, and others do so monthly.

During the cleanse period it is important to consume only organic fruits and vegetables where you can.

The Importance of Going Organic

The idea with this cleanse is that we help our body eliminate toxins. The best way to do this is to drastically reduce your exposure to toxins. By consuming only organic fruit and vegetables, we are removing a lot of the pesticides from our diet which are one of the key known carcinogens, and are found in high volumes in non-organic fruits and vegetables.

Depending on the amount, some pesticides can cause a range of adverse effects on human health such as cancer, acute/chronic injury to the nervous system, lung damage, reproductive dysfunction, as well as dysfunction of the endocrine and immune systems.

In just one (non-organic) apple there are six known or probable carcinogens, 16 suspected hormone disruptors, 5 neurotoxins and 6 developmental or reproductive toxins.

The pesticides may seem harmless because there are no immediate effects from eating them at first. However, they build up in our system over time as we consume them and often lodge in fat stores and body tissue. One of the reasons when losing weight or detoxing to make sure that your organs of elimination are working correctly!

According to the World Health Organization, every year more than

3,000,000 agriculture workers in the developing world are poisoned by pesticides, and about 18,000 of them die.

Think about the fact that pesticides are used to kill off pests. They are often found throughout every cell in the fruits, vegetables and their seeds. You can wash off the external residue of pesticides but not that which has permeated the whole fruit or vegetable

Although eating organic food will reduce your exposure to toxic pesticides and fertilisers, there is still a possibility it may sneak into the food chain. But understanding the correct foods to consume will help you to be up to six times less likely to be exposed to pesticides.

Understandably, organic produce is not affordable for everyone as it is sometimes up to 200% more expensive. Organic produce is created in smaller yields and is more labour intensive and this is what makes it much more expensive than its non-organic counterpart. If you want to lessen the cost of your organic produce, then choose from the Clean 15 List (mentioned later on). Alternatively you can save money by buying local produce or buying some healthy frozen items (this is especially good for smoothies).

If you don't have access to organic produce, the following information will be very important.

Dirty Dozen: Clean 15

Each year the Environmental Working Group (EWG) releases a "Dirty Dozen" list and "Clean 15" list. The Dirty Dozen lists the 12 most pesticide-laden fruits and vegetables (ones to always aim to buy organic). The Clean 15 provides the 15 non-organic produce least likely to be contaminated with high levels of pesticides. These are ones that you could eat, should you not be able to find organic produce.

The Dirty Dozen

Buy these organic whenever possible (Updated 2017).

- Strawberries
- Spinach
- Nectarines
- Apples
- Peaches

- Pears
- Cherries
- Grapes
- Celery
- Sweet bell peppers
- Hot Peppers
- Potatoes

The Clean 15

These are okay to buy non-organic (Updated 2017)

- Sweet Corn
- Avocados
- Pineapples
- Cabbage
- Onions
- Sweet peas frozen
- Papayas
- Asparagus
- Mangos
- Eggplant
- Honeydew Melon
- Kiwi
- Cantaloupe
- Cauliflower
- Grapefruit

CHAPTER 3

How to Cultivate Mind-set and Lifestyle Change

Accepting that we need to change and clean up our health is the first step to a complete change in mindset when it comes to regaining our overall health. For years most of us have gone along with large companies, believing that they have our best interests at heart. But most food companies are in it for the money and have no real concern for our health.

A lot of the ingredients and processes used to make store-bought food can be detrimental to our health. It may seem convenient now, but if we take the time to treat our bodies with respect then we can live a much more fulfilling life. This is much better than the odd temporary pleasures like consuming junk food.

We need to take responsibility for our health and that of our families. It has been proven, time and time again that our food and lifestyle choices are the main cause of death in the 21st century: with heart disease and cancer becoming more and more common.

But we have a choice! We can choose to take the time to educate ourselves.

I would like to take a second here to pause and congratulate you on taking this giant leap forward in your health. I am proud of you.

This new lifestyle is a complete 180-degree turn from the normal way of life for the majority of Westerners who follow the Standard American Diet (SAD). Some may meet some resistance from those around you, and that is perfectly normal. However, it is necessary for us to persevere and turn our life around if we want to achieve optimal health, especially if you or any of your loved ones is suffering from chronic illness.

CHAPTER 4

Why Smoothies, Juice and Soups?

Studies show that eating seven or more portions of fruit and vegetables each day reduces the risk of death by cancer and heart disease by up to 31%. The research also showed that vegetables have significantly higher health benefits than fruit.

Scientifically speaking, antioxidants and phytochemicals in plant foods prevent mutagenesis and carcinogenesis. Thus eating a diet rich in plant-based produce will greatly enhance your health and protect your DNA from such mutations.

Detoxing starts with your diet. By consuming only smoothies, juice and soups (made of fresh produce) we will detoxify our body. We will be eliminating processed and harmful foods. Therefore stepping out of the way of our bodies and allowing them to cleanse.

Grilling, frying, barbecuing, overcooking, browning, baking, toasting as well as the use of cooking oils like sunflower oil and linseed mutates the chemical make-up of the food we eat. Often this makes carcinogenic molecules such as acrylamide and oxygenated aldehydes, therefore increasing our risk of cancer and other diseases.

Short-term nutritional plans where we consume only liquids in the form of pure fruits, vegetables, nuts and seeds can greatly enhance detoxification.

To put it simply, by eating more fruits and vegetables you'll be filling your diet with amazing nutrients and enzymes that your body will love. This will boost your digestion and ability to fight chronic disease. The average Westerner gets over 60% of their calories from processed foods which are calorie rich and nutritionally poor, or even nutritionally empty. Consuming smoothies, juice and soups will restart your system and flood it with real superfoods.

As well as that, by having smoothies, juice and soups, you will be eliminating a lot of the food groups that are known to cause problems with our health: such as dairy, meat, processed food and fast food. Thus by doing this *Body Balance Juice Programme* you will be stepping out of your body's way to let it heal.

Let's look at each type of liquid in detail, starting with smoothies.

What Are the Health Benefits of Drinking Smoothies?

As a meal replacement, dessert or simply a brilliant addition to your health regime, smoothies are a great choice. Smoothies are great for those looking to lose weight as they are super healthy and full of vitamins and minerals, The International Journal of Obesity and Related Metabolic Disorders in 2003 found that replacing meals for healthy smoothies can safely aid in weight loss. Smoothies are rich in fruit and vegetables meaning they are packed with much-needed nutrients.

Smoothies are easy to make, as typically you can simply remove any skin/stalks and throw all of the ingredients into a blender.

One thing that is essential prior to a detox cleanse is to make sure that your organs of elimination are clear. Your colon is one of these organs. Smoothies are packed with fibre, which is great for clearing out your colon and therefore getting your body cleaned out. The fibre acts like a broom and cleans out the intestines.

Smoothies provide your body with the nutrients it needs while simultaneously giving your body much needed rest. Therefore, you will have more energy to live your life to the fullest.

Finally, you can strengthen your immune system by consuming daily smoothies. Due to the anti-inflammatory qualities of fruit and vegetables you will be giving your immune system a boost.

What you will need to create your smoothies:-

1. Smoothie maker (i.e. Nutribullet or Vitamix)
2. Air tight containers
3. Produce

Pro Smoothie Tips & Tricks

1.   Drink your smoothies immediately after making them - the earlier you drink your smoothie the more plant-based benefits it will have retained).

2.   However, if you lack time, then pack your smoothie ingredients into sealed pouches every week. Freeze the pouches and take out every evening to defrost in the fridge.

3.   Another way to do this is to make the smoothies in mason jars and freeze the jars. Placing them in the fridge each evening (to defrost) and be consumed in the morning.

N.B. Where possible it is important to consume fresh fruit and vegetables and not frozen.

CHAPTER 5

Are Soups Healthy?

Soup is soothing and especially great for colder months. The thought of all of our meals being cold and just consuming juice is not particularly appealing to everyone; this is where soup steps in. Soups allow us to eat a wide variety of vegetables in one sitting. Soup is also very filling and can be made jam-packed with vegetables. Considered as more of a meal, soup often allows you to chew your food, rather than just drink it, like with juice and smoothies.

Who doesn't love a bowl of soup? So we get to eat something here on the cleanse that is both nourishing and quite "normal". Subconsciously, we will look forward to the chance of having a nice bowl of soup at the end of the day. They are extremely soothing and make a great dinner time detox meal.

Doing a soup cleanse is often seen as an alternative to juicing. Consuming soup is quite similar to smoothies, due to the fact that it is a liquid that retains its fibre. One great benefit is that we can keep some chunks of vegetables in our soup so that we feel like we are eating. Soup is full of the good stuff and great on a detox cleanse and there is even a current trend of "soup cleanses" happening globally. However, having soups, smoothies and Juice offers variety to cleanse your body.

CHAPTER 6

Why Pure Juice Cleanse?

Fresh strained juice provides a concentrated, nutritious and dense drink. As well as giving our digestive systems a much needed rest. This allows us to use our energy for detoxification and regeneration. Especially helpful in periods of illness or during a detox cleanse. Freshly made juice is great for fasting with great health benefits.

It is generally a good idea to dilute your juice 50/50 with water. Use filtered, spring or distilled water.

How to Prepare Pre-made Juices?

It is perfectly normal to think that buying juice from the store is the same as making your own juice. However, it is really important not to consume cartons or bottles of store bought fruit juice.

Packaged fruit juice is extremely high in sugar, on top of the natural fruit sugar. This is problematic as it is not in its natural form and our bodies struggle to process foreign bodies. Store bought fruit juice has been refined so that it can keep in a package. When we consume juice from a carton then it is quite far from its life source, the life giving energy.

One way that the vital life force is lost in a packaged juice is through pasteurisation. This process kills the living enzymes leaving the juice lacking its vital life-giving enzymes and nutrients.

We all know that when we peel a fruit, it quite rapidly oxidises and turns brown. The same goes for vegetables, they either wilt or go brown when left out. So we must consume the fruit fast to gain maximum benefit. You will notice that when you make your own smoothies and juice that they lose their vibrant colour quite quickly. This does not happen to the smoothies that you buy at the store, due to the processes that they have gone through.

Getting the fruit straight from the tree is optimal. We pick the fruit and eat it or juice it – then we have a perfect situation where we can absorb the nutrients from the fruit. This is obviously not an option for most people. However, we can easily make our own smoothies and juice every day.

When we have food in containers and need to transport them around, every minute counts. Every minute the fresh fruit, vegetables, nuts or legumes are losing their vital life-giving energy. So it is of upmost importance that we make our own smoothies and juice.

From now on when we say "juice", we will be referring to fruit or vegetable juice that has been freshly prepared.

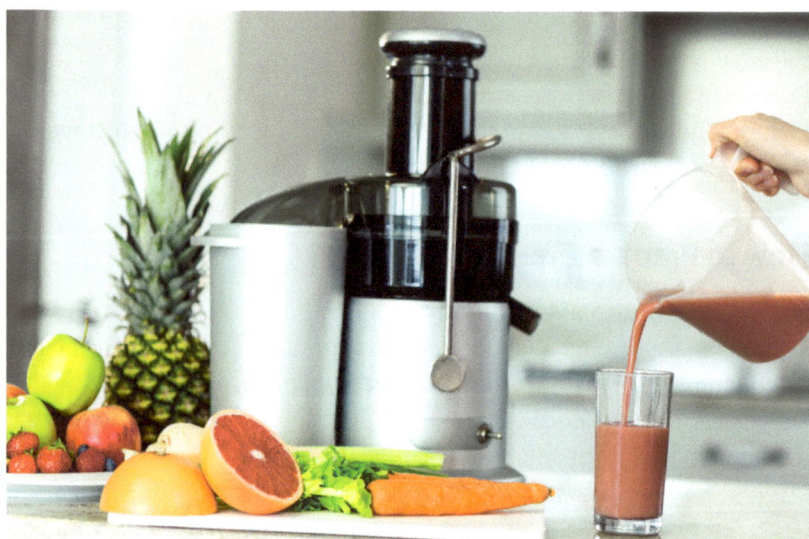

What you will need to create your juice

1. Juicer
2. Air tight containers
3. Produce

Pro tips for preparing/drinking your own fresh juice

1. Aim to drink your juice as soon as you make it. That way you will benefit from the raw food enzymes, vitamins and minerals

2.   Use a slow masticating juicer to further preserve the nutrients.

3.   The very instant you finish making and drinking your juice, rinse the cleanable parts with water. Then place the parts in a dish drainer rack until the next use.

4.   If you are working, or traveling, then you can prepare your juice for the day in an airtight container (mason jars or a thermos flask) in the morning or in the evening before and take them to work with you. Make sure that there is as little oxygen as possible in the container (as the oxygen will spoil your juice). It is best to consume your juice the minute you make it but you can store in your fridge in an airtight container for up to 48hrs if necessary (depending on the ingredients).

5.   Before getting started it is a great idea to find your local juice bar, or one near your place of work.
If you are working or travelling, it may be more difficult to keep up with your cleanse. Here are some tips for storing your fresh juice.

Pro tips for storing fresh juice

6.   Save time by making more than one juice, have some right away, and then store the rest for later.

7.   Pour into an airtight container - BPA free plastic or glass.

8.   Fill the juice up to the top of your container. This keeps your juice fresh and prevents oxidising.

9.   Store in the fridge. Juice will keep for up to 48 hours in the fridge.

10.   Freeze your juice (optional). Freeze straight away after juicing. Will keep up to a week in the freezer.

Pros and cons of juicing

Juicing is one of the best ways to get much needed essential nourishment and nutrition into your body quickly and efficiently. The juice is extracted from the produce, providing a concentrated form of nutrients. I am an advocate of juicing but let's quickly dive into the pros and cons so that we are well-informed on this mode of staying healthy.

Pros of juicing

1. Concentrated nutrients
2. Increase fruit & veg intake
3. Better nutrient absorption
4. Increased energy
5. Reduced chances of diabetes, heart disease or cancer
6. Improved and glowing skin
7. Loss of excess weight
8. Improved digestion

Cons of juicing

1. Must be organised
2. Need good juicer
3. Change of habits
4. Prep and clean-up times

When I look at it, we just need to have a great plan in place that we can follow to the letter. So get a plan from someone who has been there and done it. That is what this book is all about!

Support is also a great thing to have when you are embarking on a new journey of health. There will be people who don't understand what you are doing. Instead of trying to help you they may criticize. Therefore having a support network is always a great idea. Sometimes willpower alone is not enough, especially when life throws a curveball. So get a group of friends, family, or fellow health enthusiasts to cheer you on while you are doing your cleanse.

CHAPTER 7

Taking Control of Your Food Cravings

I f you are worried about food cravings when you are doing the *Body Balance Juice Programme* which includes soups, juice and smoothie cleanse over the next 21 days, then think again. It has been proven that food cravings are often a by-product of vitamin and mineral deficiency.

For example, people often crave chocolate when they are low in magnesium. Consuming a lot of nuts, seeds, fruits and vegetables will fill that nutritional need and reduce food cravings after you have been consuming soups, juice and smoothies.

There are other food cravings that come in the form of habitual patterns: such as, eating a pizza on a Friday (or fish and chips in some parts of the UK). Other patterns might include dining out with friends and feeling left out if you don't join.

Keep with the programme, even if just for the 21 days, and see how you feel. I have provided step by step information for you to follow, and if you stick with this programme for 21 days and see no benefits, then I will eat my hat. See if you can increase your energy, clarity, lose excess weight and improve health. It's worth a try.

If for any reason you feel you must attend an event, perhaps a wedding or special occasion that, try to opt for the healthiest food on the menu. For example, vegetable soup (without bread) or a salad. Should you need to do this for a day, then don't dwell on it. Simply make the best choice you can and get back on with the programme the following day.

CHAPTER 8

Cleaning Your Fruits and Vegetables

It is important to clean all fruits and vegetables before you eat them, to prevent food poisoning like e-coli. Bacteria can form when products are stored, therefore it is important to clean your fruit and vegetables just before you use them.

It is a good idea to buy a food produce brush to clean your vegetables. *You don't need to buy fancy vegetable cleaning products*, but there are a few tips you should follow to make sure your fruits and vegetables are clean and safe to eat.

Soak fresh fruits and vegetables in water with apple cider vinegar for 15 minutes to remove bacteria and pesticides from the surface.

What you will need:

1. A big tub to soak your fruits and vegetables
2. Apple cider vinegar

CHAPTER 9

Fast Food -vs-
Processed Food

It is a fact that the average Westerner eats too much of everything. So you will probably save money during your detox cleanse, just by cutting back on unnecessary snacks and pre packed goods: no packaged lunches or snacks. There will be no eating out for the 21 days and your wallet may very well thank you.

Eating fast food on a regular basis can lead to obesity due to the amount of calories, fat, and sodium in fast food meals. Not to mention the additional problems like high blood pressure, high cholesterol and dental distress.

When we talk about "processed food", we are referring to food products that are created using commercial practices like the adding of artificial food colouring, food additives, irradiation and preservatives. Most processed foods have several additives which are more toxic when combined. For example, when food dyes mix with MSG then we have a stronger toxic compound created. Many of the food colourings have been linked to a wide array of health problems, from hyperactivity to tumours.

Most fast food and processed foods contain harmful chemicals and preservatives. Processed foods also contain trans-fats in the form of partially hydrogenated oil which is a key an ingredient in packaged foods, such as crisps, crackers, pies, cookies or cakes. Such trans-fats are linked to shortened lifespans and heart disease. Aluminum can be found in sweets and foods that need raising agents. Aluminum is toxic to humans and builds up over time negatively affecting our brain and nervous systems.

By cutting out processed and fast food by crowding them out with soups, smoothies and juice, we will be nourishing our bodies from the inside out.

Interesting Facts

Mercury is the second most toxic metal on the planet.

Did you know that high fructose corn syrup (HFCS) is used extensively in processed and fast food and has mercury in it? Not just that, the process to create HFCS starts with soaking corn in mercury.

CHAPTER 10

What to Expect

For the first day or two of a fast, your body uses up the food remaining in your digestive tract from previous meals. For the next couple of days, your body uses stored food reserves from your liver. This means that an effective fast doesn't really begin until about the *fifth day, so stick with it.* After the third day things will be easier. By the time you reach the fifth day – you will start to feel your body lighter and clearer.

Cleansing Reactions

Cleansing reactions are undesirable (but temporary). *Detox Symptoms:* when detoxing you may have some negative side effects, such as body aches, headaches, nausea, nasal congestion, sore throat, constipation, diarrhoea, skin rashes, or flu-like symptoms. This is perfectly normal.

There are a few reasons that you may experience some of these detox symptoms. One reason for the side effects is because your body stores toxins inside fat cells. These fat cells become inflamed to protect you from toxic exposure. When detoxing, these fat cells will shrink and die, therefore releasing the toxic chemicals into your body.

Other reasons for cleansing reactions can be due to your organs of elimination being blocked or the dying off of unhealthy bacteria.

Six Great Tips for Lessening Cleansing Reactions

It is a good idea to protect yourself and do as much as you can to avoid some of these symptoms. There are a few things that you can do to protect yourself and help your body detox. These include;

1. Dry skin brushing
2. Bathing in Epsom salts
3. Castor oil packs on your liver.
4. Supplements that help with cleansing reactions such as activated charcoal and magnesium supplements
5. Sauna/Steam Room
6. Keep active: go for walks, do light yoga or jump on a rebounder

CHAPTER 11

Buying Produce for Your Programme

You can always shop at your local supermarket if they provide organic produce. However you will find that the majority of the store is off limits. This becomes quite interesting when we think about the global health crisis in the world right now. I would suggest ordering your produce online where possible to make sure that you don't get tempted by the products that you usually buy in the shops.

Buy Local

As I mentioned before, you can save money, reduce your carbon footprint, and help local businesses by buying from local farmers or farmers markets. Some areas also have box schemes that you can buy into that allow you to have a delivery of fresh, local, organic produce. These are often dropped off at local hotspots or delivered straight to your door.

Fruit/Vegetable Picking

You can get involved with fruit and vegetable picking at local farms which can be fun and allow you to stock up on more local fruits and vegetables than you would normally see in a shop.

Grow Your Own

If you have a small garden, you can create raised beds, use containers or grow produce that works well in your season and area. This is the best possible way to obtain real fresh, living nutrition. Growing our own produce is a very rewarding process that will provide you with optimal enzymes and nutrition. If you don't have space, then you can get involved with a community garden or rent a plot.

Frozen fruits and Vegetables

It is often easier to stock up on frozen fruits and vegetables. Where I live for example, it is easy to go to the local eco store and buy frozen organic berries all year round. However, if you wanted to buy them fresh they would need to have been flown into the country (when not in season locally).

See page 33 for your shopping list

CHAPTER 12

How to Eliminate Inflammation

While on this diet you will be eliminating all inflammatory foods like: dairy, fish and meat which significantly reduces the risk of cancer. Fruits and vegetables are anti-inflammatory and provide a huge amount of nutrition. The benefits of whole fruit and vegetables are numerous: from boosting your immune system, stabilising blood sugars (therefore curbing diabetes) to improving cardiovascular health.

Alkaline vs Acidic Foods

When we metabolise foods they leave a residue and this residue (often referred to as ash) is either acidic, neutral or alkaline. This ash is then filtered through our kidneys and organs of elimination to be removed from the body. Diseases like cancer thrive in an acidic environment and also create more acidity with its waste.

The pH scale measures how acidic or alkaline a substance is. The pH scale ranges from 0 to 14.

Therefore, a lot of people believe that a more alkaline body equals better health. Below is a quick overview of foods and their pH.

Acidic: (pH 0-7) alcohol, dairy, eggs, grains, fish, and meat

Neutral: (pH 7) natural fats, starches and sugars.

Alkaline: (pH 7-14) fruit, nuts, legumes and vegetables.

There are a variety of views surrounding the acid/alkaline food debate (as there are with nutrition in general). However nobody can deny that eating a lot of fruit, vegetables and healthy plant foods, while refraining processed junk foods is good for your health. The most alkaline foods are green drinks or salads, containing foods like: celery, kale, parsley, spinach and avocado.

CHAPTER 13

Let's Start 21-Day Body Balance Juice Programme!

Before we get started, below is a shopping list for you to purchase your produce and to ensure you have all the items required for the *Body Balance Juice Programme*. With the 21 days menus it's a guide to your health freedom.

NB: You may need to review your weekly produces after week one to ensure you have all the produce required for this programme.

Body Balance Juice Programme -Shopping List

ITEM	QUANTITY	ITEM	QUANTITY
Asparagus	6	Avocado	3
Baby Spinach Leaves	2 Packs	Banana	3
Bean Sprouts	1 Pack	Beetroot	1 Pack
Beetroot With Leaves	6	Blackcurrant	1 Pack
Blueberries	2 Packs	Broccoli	1
Butternut Squash	1	Cabbage	1
Carrots	13	Cauliflower	1

Celery	3 Packs	Cherries	1 Pack
Chicory Leaves	1 Pack	Coriander	1 Pack
Courgette	1 Pack	Cucumber	6
Fennel	2	Fresh Lychees	15
Garlic	1	Ginger	2
Grapefruit	4	Green Apple	8
Green Cabbage	1	Green Pepper	2
Horseradish	1	Kale	1 Pack
Kiwi	4	Large Tomato	2
Leek	4	Lemon	12
Lemon Thyme	1	Lime	12
Lovage	1 Pack	Mango	2
Mint	1 Pack	Nectarine	4
Okra	1 Pack	Onions	6
Orange	4	Parsley	1 Pack
Parsnip	6	Passion Fruit	4
Papaya	2	Peach	4
Pear	4	Pineapple	1
Pink Apple	6	Pistachios	1 Bag
Pomegranate	2	Pumpkin	1

Quinoa	250G	Raspberries	2 Packs
Red Apple	1	Red Cabbage	1
Red Grapes	1 Pack	Red Or Green Chillies	2
Red Pepper	2	Red Plum	4
Red Radish	1 Pack	Rocket Leaves	1 Pack
Romaine Lettuce Leaves	1 Pack	Satsuma	4
Shelled Peas	2 Bags	Spring Onions	1 Bunch
Sweet Potatoes	4	Swiss Card Leaf	1 Pack
Watercress	1 Pack	Watermelon	1

ADDITIONAL PRODUCTS			
Almond Milk	Almonds	Apple Cider Vinegar	Aloe Vera Juice
Avocado Oil	Bay Leaves	Black Pepper Corns	Chia Seeds
Cinnamon	Coconut Water	Coconut Cream	Coconut Milk
Dried Fruits	Dried Wild Mushrooms	Elderflower Tea	Flaxseeds
Himalayan Salt	Hemp Seeds	Honey	Nutmeg
Rolled Oats	Olive Oil	Pumpkin Seeds	Sesame Seeds
Spirulina	Stevia Leaves	Turmeric	Walnuts

DAY 1

Breakfast
Pure Juice

Lunch
Broccoli Green Cleanser

Dinner
Vegetable Soup

Extra Boost
Lime & Broccoli Shot

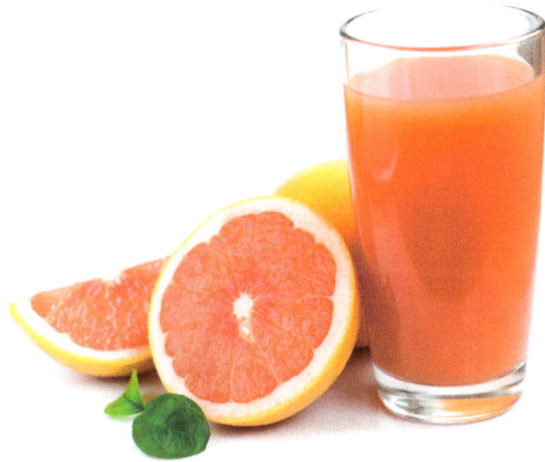

Pure Juice

½ grapefruit   2 stalks celery

1 lemon   ½ cucumber

3 red radishes   2 cm root ginger

1 red apple

Wash all produce. Peel Grapefruit & lemon. Core apple. Cut all produce size (to fit in a juicer). Juice then pour.
o a smoothie maker.

FOOD	NUTRITIONAL BENEFITS
Grapefruit	Maintain a healthy heart and blood pressure
Lemon	Anti-parasitic, alkalizing all round cleanser
Radishes	Purify blood, cleanse liver and stomach.
Apple	Cleanse colon, regulate blood sugar, lower cholesterol
Celery	Rich in antioxidants and beneficial enzymes
Cucumber	Stress relief, hydration, skin health
Ginger	Powerful anti-inflammatory (good for arthritis), soothes the stomach

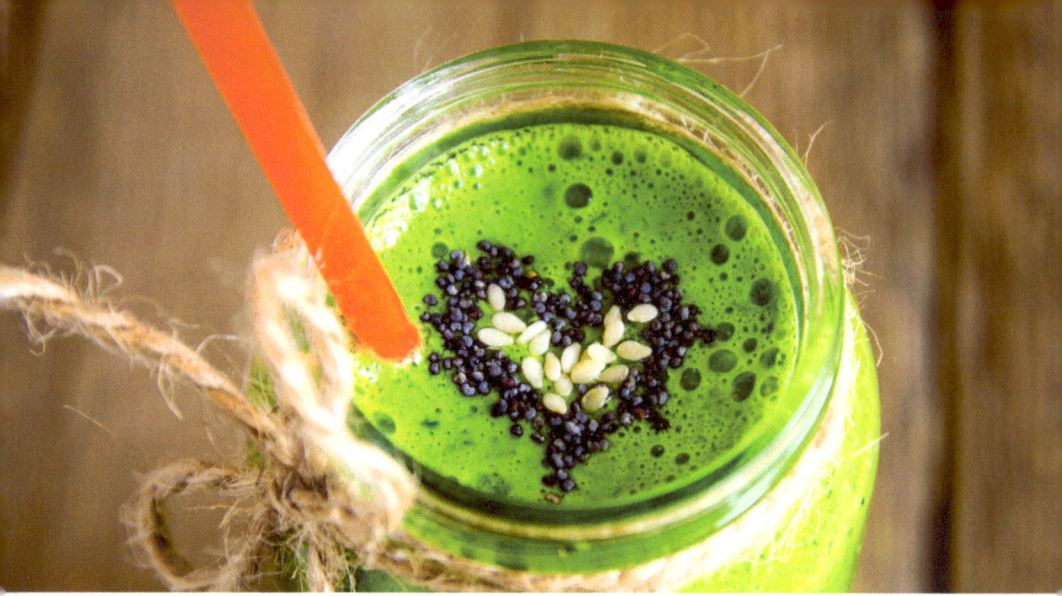

Broccoli Green Cleanser

4 stems broccoli

1 cucumber   1 carrot

1 lime   3 celery stalks

Small bunch of parsley   A handful of baby spinach leaves

1 teaspoon chia seeds, flaxseeds, pumpkin or avocado oil to serve

Wash all produce. Peel Lime. Juice greens first, so that the other fruits will push the greens through. Cut all produce to size (to fit in a juicer). Juice then pour

FOOD	NUTRITIONAL BENEFITS
Cucumber	Stress relief, hydration, skin health
Lime	Cleanses blood, improves digestion and great for thyroid health.
Celery	Rich in antioxidants and beneficial enzymes
Spinach	Superfood, nutrient-rich - skin, hair and bone health
Carrot	Rich in beta-carotene: for healthy skin, immune system & eye health
Parsley	Good for kidney and bladder health. Cleanses & relieves constipation
Flaxseed	Heart Healthy. Omega 2 rich. Lubricates joints.
Chia Seeds	Rich in Omeg-3 fatty acids, antioxidants, fibre, iron and calcium. Also helps raise HDL cholesterol, good cholesterol that finds against heart attack and stroke.
Pumpkin Seed	Contains phytosterols and free radical scavenging antitoxins. Rich in magnesium, manganese, copper, protein and zinc
Broccoli	Builds collagen - forms tissue and bone. Antioxidant.

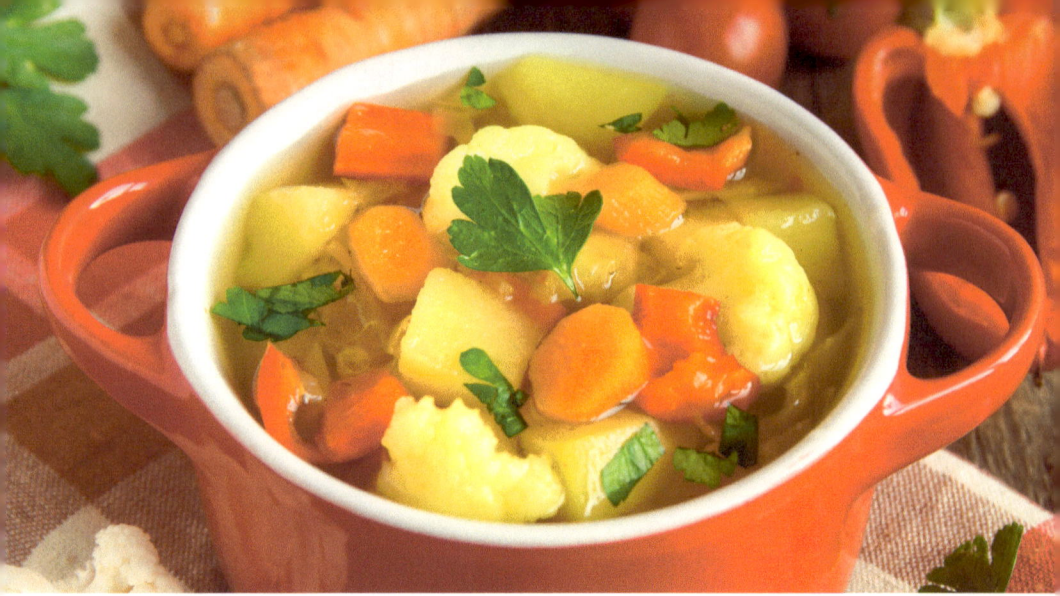

Vegetable Soup

3 cloves garlic

1 bay leaf

Small bunch of parsley

2 onions

Floret of cauliflower

1 leek

2 sweet potatoes

1 parsnip

3 carrots

2 litres water

Himalayan salt to taste

1. Put 2 litres of water on to boil
2. Wash all vegetables
3. Peel and dice onion – add to water
4. Peel Garlic and crush – add to water
5. Chop ends off leek and cut
6. Peel and chop parsnips, carrots and sweet potatoes – add to pot

FOOD	NUTRITIONAL BENEFITS
Garlic	Neutralize free radicals preventing cellular damage.
Bay leaf	Antibacterial and anti-fungal properties. Soothes body aches
Cauliflower	Good source of Vitamin C, K, protein, riboflavin, niacin, magnesium, thiamine, phosphorous, potassium, fibre, vitamin B6, folate, pantothenic acid, and manganese
Parsley	Good for kidney and bladder health. Cleanses & relieves constipation
Onions	Balance blood sugar. Cancer-fighting.
Leek	Fight free radicals in your body. Anti-cancer. Anti-diabetes.
Parsnip	High in potassium: Reduce blood pressure. Improve heart health.
Sweet potato	Super food. Good for diabetes. Anti-cancer. Immune system booster.
Carrots	Rich in beta-carotene: for healthy skin, immune system & eye health
Himalayan salt	Balance pH and blood sugar. Detoxify body, improves hydration.

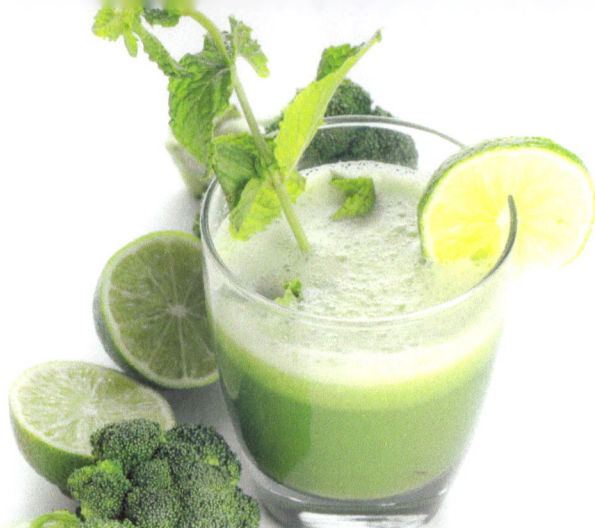

Lime & Broccoli Shot

1 broccoli floret   250 ml water

1 lime

With 250 ml water add lime and broccoli to a smoothie maker. Drink this shot mid-morning or mid-afternoon

FOOD	NUTRITIONAL BENEFITS
Lime	Improves digestion, reduced respiratory and urinary disorder, relief constipation and treatment of scurvy, piles, peptic ulcer gout and gums. Weight loss. Aids skin and eyes
Broccoli	Builds collagen - forms tissue and bone. Antioxidant.

DAY 2

Breakfast
Lemon, Grapefruit and Lime Juice

Lunch
Beetroot Juice

Dinner
Minestrone Soup

Extra Boost
Cranberry, Coconut and Chia Blast

Lemon, Grapefruit and Lime Juice

1 lemon	250 ml
1 pink grapefruit	1 sprig of mint
1 lime	1 teaspoon honey or 2 stevia leaves (powder)

Wash all produce. Peel lemon, grapefruit and lime. Cut all produce size (to fit in a juicer). Juice then pour. Add honey or stevia to taste

FOOD	NUTRITIONAL BENEFITS
Lemon	Anti-parasitic, alkalizing all round cleanser
Grapefruit	Maintain a healthy heart and blood pressure
Lime	Cleanses blood, improves digestion and great for thyroid health.
Honey	Anti-bacterial, anti-fungal. Helps prevent cancer and heart disease.

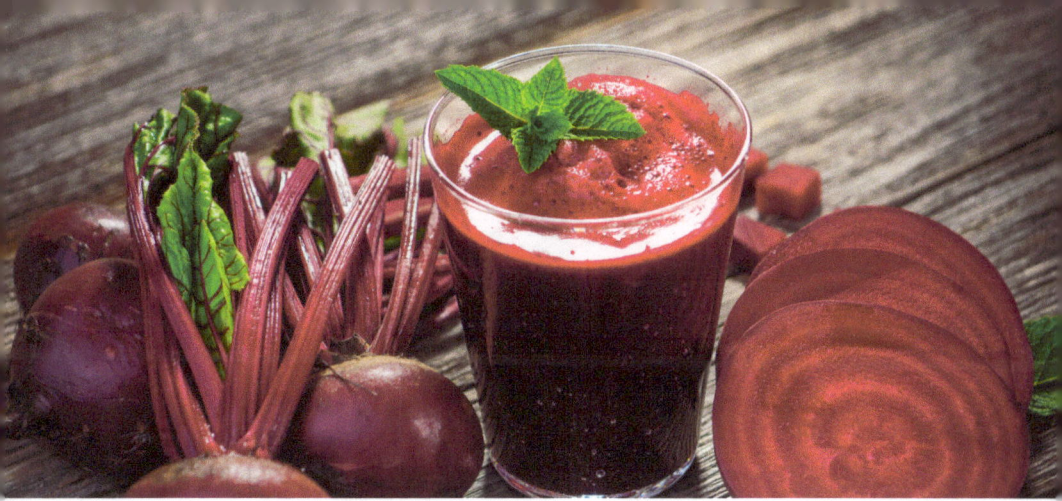

Beetroot Juice

2 cm piece of ginger root

1 beetroot and 3 beetroot leaves

1 orange

1 teaspoon walnut, almond or olive oil

½ lime

Wash all produce. Peel orange. Cut all produce size (to fit in a juicer). Juice then pour.

FOOD	NUTRITIONAL BENEFITS
Beetroot	Amazing for blood & liver health. Increases oxygen in the blood.
Orange	Anti-diabetes, skin food, heart healthy, anti-cancer, vitamin c rich
Ginger	Powerful anti-inflammatory (good for arthritis), soothes the stomach
Walnut	Rich in ALA - good for the brain, anti-inflammatory
Almond	Relieves Stress. May prevent cardiovascular disease.

Minestrone Soup

3 carrots

2 onions

2 stalks celery

1 leek

2 potatoes

1 parsnip or sweet potato

Bunch of spring onions

150 g fresh or frozen shelled peas

Parsley leaves

Wash produce. Peel and dice onions. Peel and chop carrots, potato, parsnip and sweet potato. Chop celery and leek. Place all ingredients in the pot. Bring all vegetables to boil.

FOOD	NUTRITIONAL BENEFITS
Food	Nutritional Benefits
Carrots	Rich in beta carotene: for healthy skin, immune system & eye health
Onions	Balance blood sugar. Cancer fighting.
Celery	Rich in antioxidants and beneficial enzymes
Leek	Fight free radicals in your body. Anti-cancer. Anti-diabetes.
Potato	Anti-cancer. Supports heart health.
Parsnip	High in potassium: Reduce blood pressure. Improve heart health.
Sweet potato	Super food. Good for diabetes. Anti-cancer. Immune system booster.
Spring onion	Lowers blood sugar, heart healthy, anti-bacterial
Peas	Immune system booster, antioxidant, anti-inflammatory
Parsley	Good for kidney and bladder health. Cleanses & relieves constipation

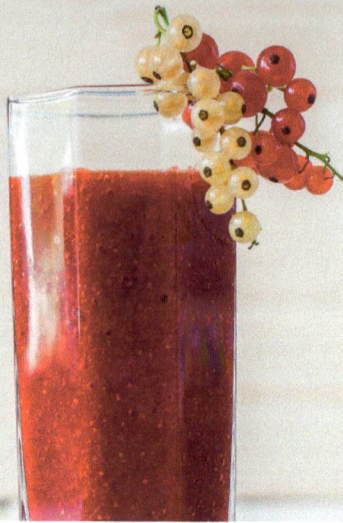

Cranberry, Coconut and Chia Blast

2 tablespoons chia seeds

50 g cranberries

50 g strawberries

125 ml water

125 ml coconut water

Wash all produce. Place all ingredients in the smoothie maker and blend - then pour.

FOOD	NUTRITIONAL BENEFITS
Chia Seeds	Heart-healthy, prevents stroke, rich in nutrients
Raspberries	Antioxidant-rich, fight cancer, anti-aging
Cranberry	Relief from UTI unary tract infection. Respiratory discomfort
Coconut Water	Hydration. Electrolytes. Antioxidant.

DAY 3

Having headaches or feeling tired is normal!

Breakfast
Mango & Quinoa Porridge with Pomegranate,
Pistachios & Dried Fruits

Lunch
Energy Green Juice

Dinner
Minestrone Green Soup

Extra Boost
Cherries Crush

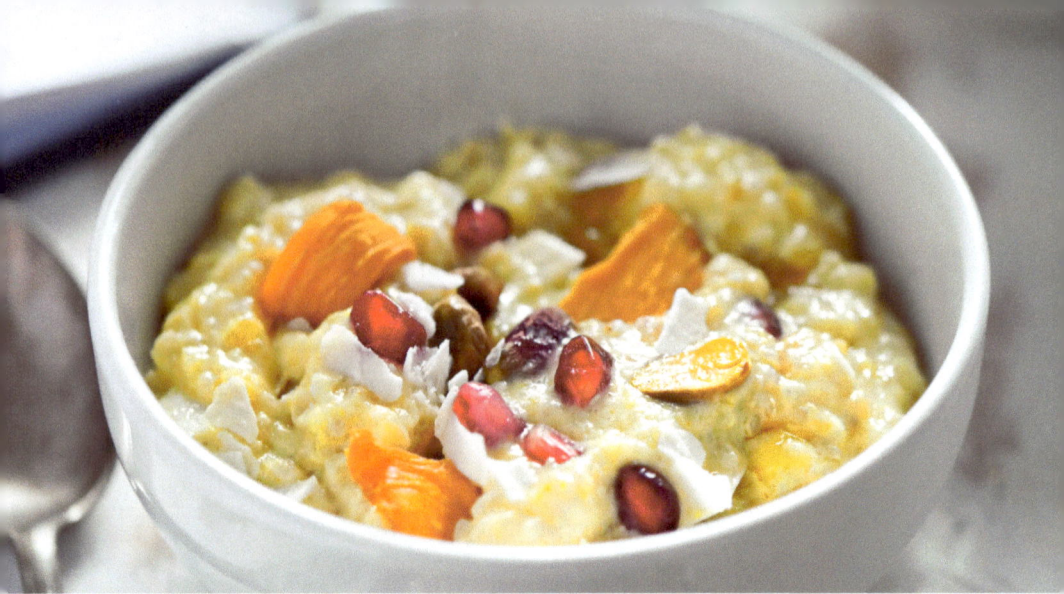

Mango & Quinoa Porridge with Pomegranate, Pistachios & Dried Fruits

250 ml almond milk

140 g quinoa

1 small mango

15 pomegranates

10 pistachios

Hand full of dry fruits

About 4 cm cinnamon powder

Peel and chop mango. Blend mango until smooth. Add the quinoa, almond milk and cinnamon to simmer for 3 minutes. Add to mango and blend. Add pistachios, pomegranate and dried fruits

FOOD	NUTRITIONAL BENEFITS
Almond Milk	Relieves Stress. May prevent cardiovascular disease.
Mango	Good for skin, eye health, prevent cancer, alkalizes body
Cinnamon	Fights diabetes, antioxidant-rich, heart healthy, improves brain function
Pomegranate	Promotes cardiovascular health, blood pressure. Good source of fibre, contains vitamins E, A, C, Iron and other antioxidants
Pistachio	Promotes healthy gut bacteria, lower blood sugar, high in protein, antioxidants, lower cholesterol and helps weight loss
Quinoa	Contains iron, lysine, Riboflavin (B2), manganese, magnesium, high in fibre

Energy Green Juice

Handful of Kale

½ lime

1 green apple

3 green cabbage leaves

Handful bean sprouts

Handful of baby spinach

Ice cubes (optional)

Core apple, peel lime. Add all ingredients to smoothie maker and blend well together.

FOOD	NUTRITIONAL BENEFITS
Kale	High in iron, zero fat, prevent cancer, anti-inflammatory
Lime	Cleanses blood, improves digestion and great for thyroid health.
Apple	Cleanse colon, regulate blood sugar, lower cholesterol
Green cabbage	Fights inflammation, promotes healthy gut, combats chronic disease
Bean sprouts	High in vitamin c and folic acid. Protein source.
Spinach	Super food, nutrient rich - skin, hair and bone health

Minestrone Green Soup

Minestrone soup (reminder of day two soup)

2 handfuls of spinach leaves

Fresh nutmeg

Heat soup and bring to boil then add spinach leaves and nutmeg (transfer soup to a blender or smoothie machine for 10 minutes.).

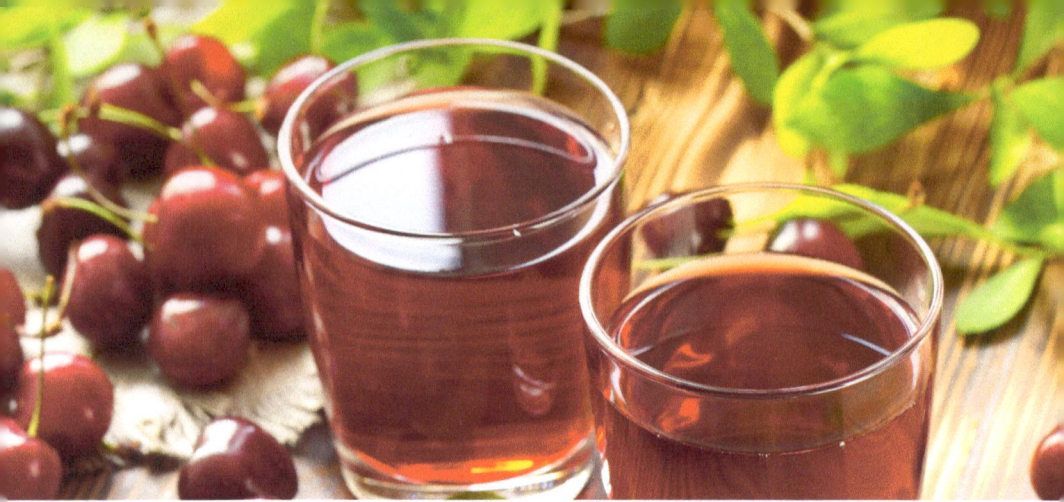

Cherries Crush

50 g cherries

1 small green or pink apple

125 ml water

Wash produce. Remove stone from cherries and chop in pieces; Core apple. Put all ingredients in a juicer machine

FOOD	NUTRITIONAL BENEFITS
Cherries	Arthritis pain relief, reduce belly fat, reduce inflammation and your risk of gout, cancer-preventative compounds
Apple	Cleanse colon, regulate blood sugar, lower cholesterol

DAY 4

Nuts and seeds are rich in good fats and amino acids.

Breakfast
Banana, Seed and Nut Milk

Lunch
Fully Loaded Greens

Dinner
Wild Mushroom and Cauliflower Chowder

Extra Boost
Aloe Vera and Lychee Cooler

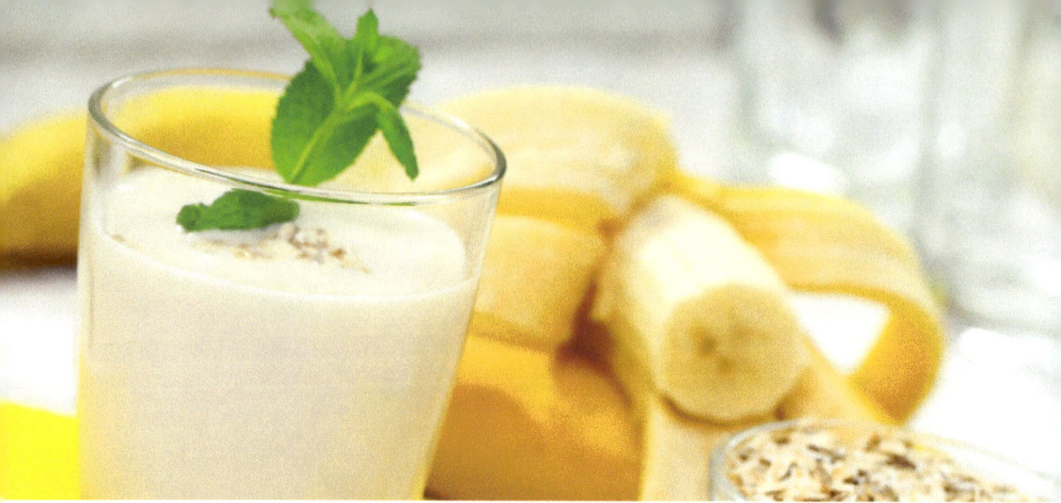

Banana, Seed and Nut Milk

12 almonds

1 banana (slices to serve)

1 tablespoon sesame seeds

2 tablespoons sunflower or pumpkin seeds

2 tablespoons flaxseeds

Rolled oats

350 ml water

Heat water and pour over the nuts and seeds and leave for 10 minutes. Pour the whole mixture in a blender. Place the banana slices over the top

FOOD	NUTRITIONAL BENEFITS
Almonds	Relieves Stress. May prevent cardiovascular disease.
Banana	Fibre rich, ease digestion, prevent anaemia
Sesame Seeds	Bone health, beat diabetes, ease digestion, reduce inflammation
Flaxseeds	Heart Healthy. Omega 2 rich. Lubricates joints.
Sunflower seeds	Heart-healthy, antioxidant, good for thyroid health and mood.
Pumpkin seeds	A nutritional powerhouse, good for nerves, antioxidant, protein-rich
Oats	Constipation relief, antioxidant-rich, protects skin, lowers blood sugar.

Fully Loaded Greens

6 sprigs of watercress

1 green apple

6 chicory leaves

1 swiss chard leaf

3 red cabbage leaves

½ green pepper

3 romaine lettuce leaves

3 beetroots leaves

1 handful of kale

Core apple. Discard any pips or core. Remove the stalk from the chard leaf. Juice the greens first before the pepper and apple.

FOOD	NUTRITIONAL BENEFITS
Watercress	Protects against cancer, antioxidant, bone & teeth strength.
Apple	Cleanse colon, regulate blood sugar, cholesterol
Chicory leafs	A great all-round detoxifier, antibacterial, prevents heartburn
Beetroot leafs	Amazing for blood & liver health. Increases oxygen in the blood.
Romaine lettuce	Fight free radicals, bone strength, eye health
Swiss chard	A nutritional powerhouse, assist calcium transportation & healing
Red cabbage	Fights inflammation, promotes a healthy gut, combats chronic disease
Green pepper	Anti-inflammatory, multiple health benefits. Protects against cancer.
Kale	High in iron, zero fat, prevent cancer, anti-inflammatory

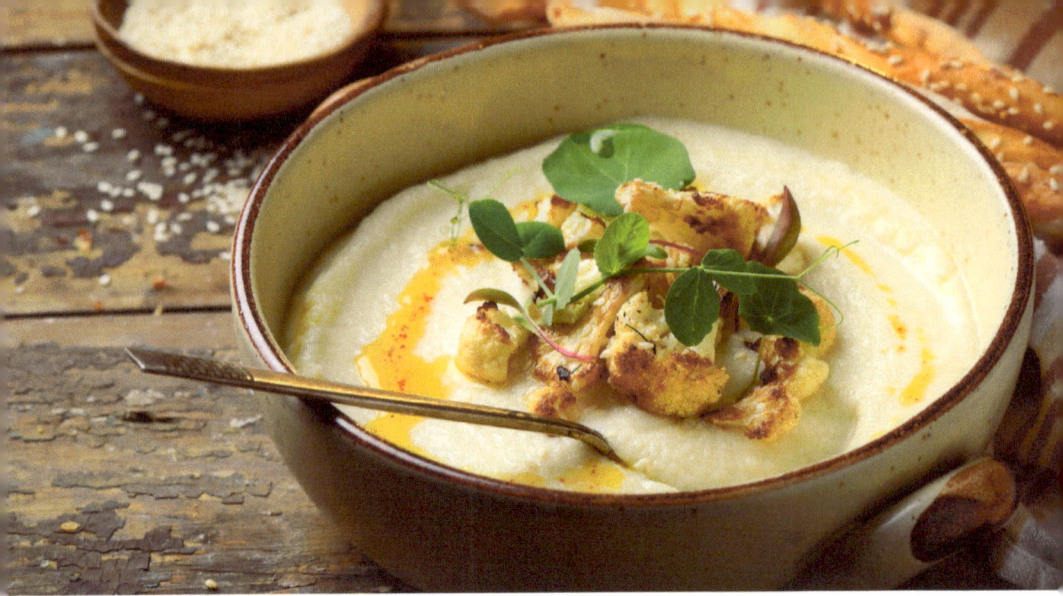

Wild Mushroom and Cauliflower Chowder

1 leek

2 stalks celery

1 cauliflower

Handful of coriander

250 ml vegetable tea (see Day One)

Handful of dried wild mushrooms

1. Cut mushrooms in half
2. Place in a bowl and pour boiling water.
3. Leave to soak for 15 minutes.
4. Cut cauliflower,
5. Chop stalks of coriander finely,
6. Add chopped celery and leek in a pan
7. Bring to boil and simmer for 20 minutes.
8. Drain, keeping all the liquid.
9. Add mushrooms and soaking liquid to a clean pan with the vegetable tea and cauliflower liquid.
10. Heat mixture (5 minutes)
11. Serve in a soup bowl.

FOOD	NUTRITIONAL BENEFITS
Leek	Fight free radicals in your body. Anti-cancer. Anti-diabetes.
Celery	Rich in antioxidants and beneficial enzymes
Cauliflower	Help fight cancer, balance hormones, heart healthy
Wild mushrooms	Vitamin D rich - essential for every system in the body.
Coriander	Cleansing, reduce infections, lower blood sugars

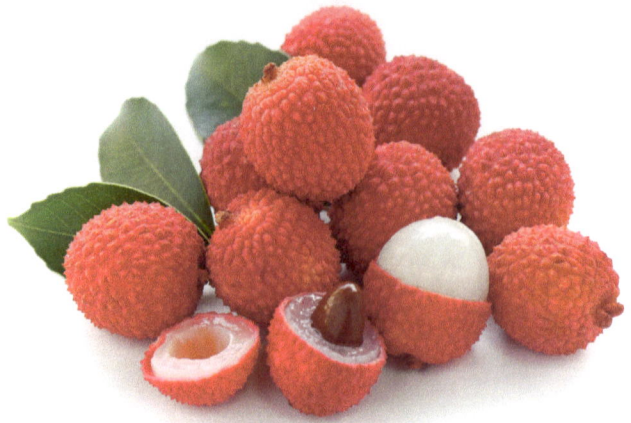

Aloe Vera and Lychee Chiller

250 ml aloe vera juice

Eight fresh lychees

Cold water

Peel the lychees and remove stones. Put in a blender with aloe vera juice

FOOD	NUTRITIONAL BENEFITS
Aloe vera juice	Heartburn relief, good for life, increase hydration, alkaline
Lychees	Boosts immune system, good for skin, improve digestion, anti-cancer

DAY 5

Absorbing nutrients more easily with appropriate gut flora.

Breakfast
Pear & Sweet Potato Boost

Lunch
Avocado, Spinach and Spirulina Smoothie

Dinner
Potassium Broth

Extra Boost
Lime, Plum and Elderflower Chiller

Pear and Sweet Potato Boost

1 pear

1 carrot

1 small sweet potato

3 romaine lettuce leaves

1 grapefruit

½ fennel bulb

Peel grapefruit. Chop and peel the sweet potato, carrot and pear. Place all ingredients in a juicer.

FOOD	NUTRITIONAL BENEFITS
Pear	Calms nerves, supple joints, and good for gout/arthritis. Mild laxative.
Carrot	Rich in beta carotene: for healthy skin, immune system & eye health
Sweet potato	Super food. Good for diabetes. Anti-cancer. Immune system booster.
Romaine lettuce	Fight free radicals, bone strength, eye health
Grapefruit	Maintain a healthy heart and blood pressure
Fennel	Cleansing benefits, rich in vitamin B6, antioxidant rich, calcium rich
Lettuce	Helps with sleep and anxiety, prevents cancer

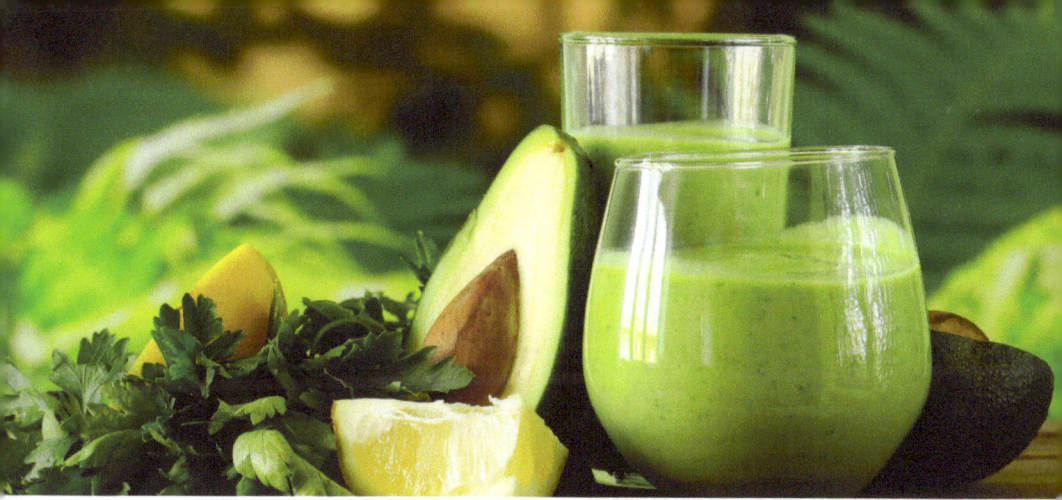

Avocado, Spinach and Spirulina Smoothie

½ teaspoon spirulina

1 small avocado

1 banana

3 sprigs of mint

150 g spinach

1 lemon

1 orange

1 teaspoon honey

or 2 stevia leaves

Wash produce. Peel lemon, banana and orange. Remove stone from avocado. Whizz all ingredients in a smoothie machine.

FOOD	NUTRITIONAL BENEFITS
Spirulina	Super food, iron & protein rich, particularly great for the blood.
Avocado	Fibre rich, heart healthy, brain healthy, good for nervous system
Mint	Aids in digestion. Antiseptic, antibacterial, helps IBS & headaches
Spinach	Super food, nutrient rich-skin, hair, bone health
Lemon	Anti-parasitic, alkalizing all round cleanser
Orange	Anti-diabetes, skin food, heart healthy, anti-cancer, vitamin c rich
Banana	Fibre rich, ease digestion, prevent anaemia
Honey	Anti-bacterial, anti-fungal. Helps prevent cancer and heart disease.
Stevia	No calories, anti-cancer, good for diabetes.

Potassium Consommé

1 litre water	1 celery stalk
4 carrots	Small bunch of parsley
1 onion	Handful of spinach 1 leek
1 leek	

1. *Prepare the vegetables*
2. *Bring water to boil.*
3. *Dice celery and carrots.*
4. *Remove root from the end of leek (discard) and slice into rings.*
5. *Transfer all the ingredients into a blender until smooth.*
6. *Add salt to taste.*

FOOD	NUTRITIONAL BENEFITS
Carrots	Rich in beta-carotene: for healthy skin, immune system & eye health
Onion	Balance blood sugar. Cancer-fighting.
Leek	Fight free radicals in your body. Anti-cancer. Anti-diabetes.
Celery	Rich in antioxidants and beneficial enzymes
Parsley	Good for kidney and bladder health. Cleanses & relieves constipation
Spinach	Superfood, nutrient-rich - skin, hair and bone health

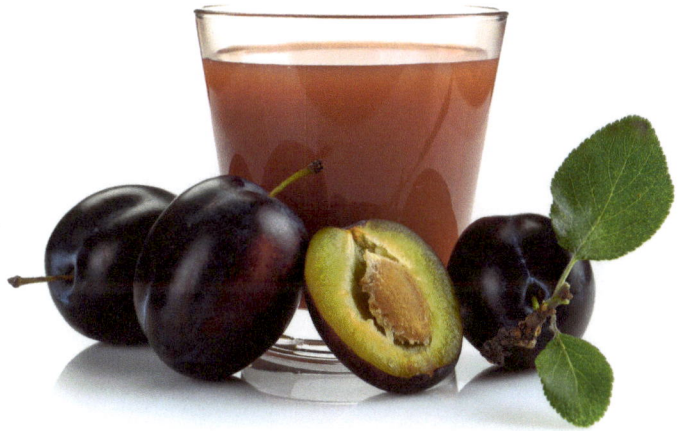

Plum Chiller

2 red plums

1 lime

2 sprigs of mint

500ml elderflower tea or juice

Cut plum in half and remove stone. Peel lime, cut into chunks and remove any pips. Place all ingredients in a blender with tea (or juice) and whizz for one minute

FOOD	NUTRITIONAL BENEFITS
Plums	Vitamin C rich, great for constipation/ IBS.
Lime	Cleanses blood, improves digestion and great for thyroid health.
Mint	Aids in digestion. Antiseptic, antibacterial, helps IBS & headaches
Elderflower	Good for constipation, relieve flu and cold, increase sweating, cleansing

DAY 6

Rainbow day (colours) will give you nutritional benefit. Each of the colours of fruits and vegetables is great for different jobs. For example: Orange food is great for skin and eye health.

Breakfast
Cucumber, Watermelon and Celery Juice

Lunch
Rhumba Smoothie

Dinner
Beetroot and Cabbage Broth

Extra Boost
Pineapple Pina Colada

Cucumber, Watermelon and Celery Juice

⅛ watermelon

½ Cucumber

1 sprig of mint

3 stalks of celery

1 Lemon

Cut cucumber and watermelon into slices and place in a juicer. Put mint leaves in the juicer.

FOOD	NUTRITIONAL BENEFITS
Cucumber	Stress relief, hydration, skin health
Watermelon	Increase blood flow. Immune System Support.
Mint	Aids in digestion. Antiseptic, antibacterial, helps IBS & headaches
Lemon	Improves digestion, freshens breath, skin. Good source of vitamin C. Helps prevents kidney stones
Celery	Rich in antioxidants and beneficial enzymes

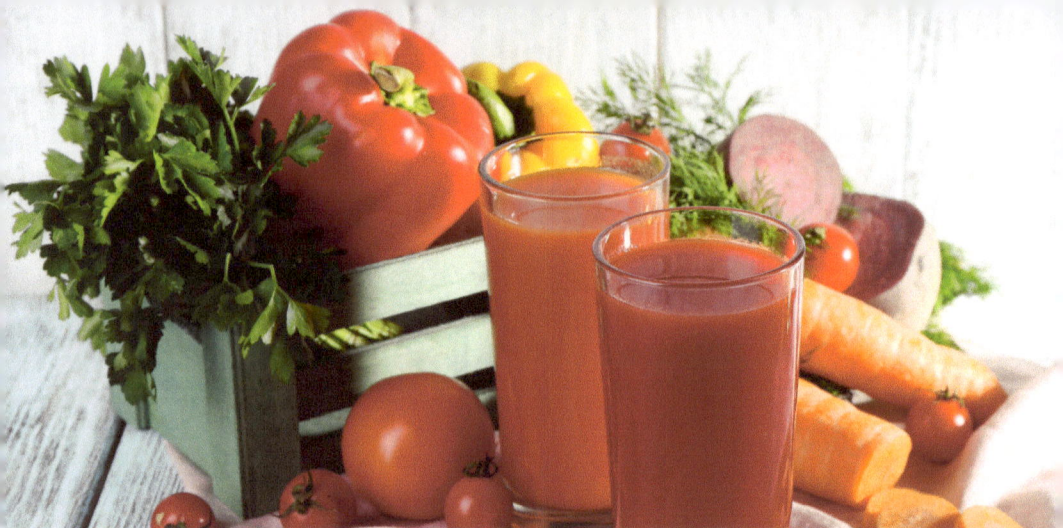

Rhumba Smoothie

1 large tomato	2 carrots
½ cucumber	1 red and yellow sweet pepper
1 celery stalk, with leaves	1 teaspoon apple cider vinegar
1 fresh red or green chili (2cm)	Add Himalayan salt to taste
1 tablespoon olive oil	2 stems of coriander
1 small avocado	500 ml water
1 beetroot	

Peel and stone avocado. Cut tomato, sweet peppers, beetroot, carrots, cucumber, celery, red chili and lemon in chunks. Chop coriander. Place all ingredients in a smoothie machine.

FOOD	NUTRITIONAL BENEFITS
Tomato	Antioxidant, anti-cancer, eye health, digestive comfort, manage diabetes
Cucumber	Stress relief, hydration, skin health
Celery	Rich in antioxidants and beneficial enzymes
Chilli	Cleanse sinus, aids digestion, relieve migraine & muscle pain
Olive oil	Antioxidant-rich, anti-inflammatory, prevent strokes, heart healthy
Avocado	Fiber-rich, heart healthy, brain healthy, good for the nervous system
Beetroot	Good source of Iron and folate. Helps to lower blood pressure, boost exercise performance and prevent dementia
Carrot	Rich in beta-carotene: for healthy skin, immune system & eye health
Apple cider vinegar	Cleansing, Regulates blood sugar, improves skin, boosts gut health
Sweet pepper	Rich in vitamin C, beta-carotene, antioxidant, anti-inflammatory, phytochemicals
Himalayan salt	Balance pH and blood sugar. Detoxify body. Improves hydration.
Coriander	Cleansing, reduce infections, lower blood sugars

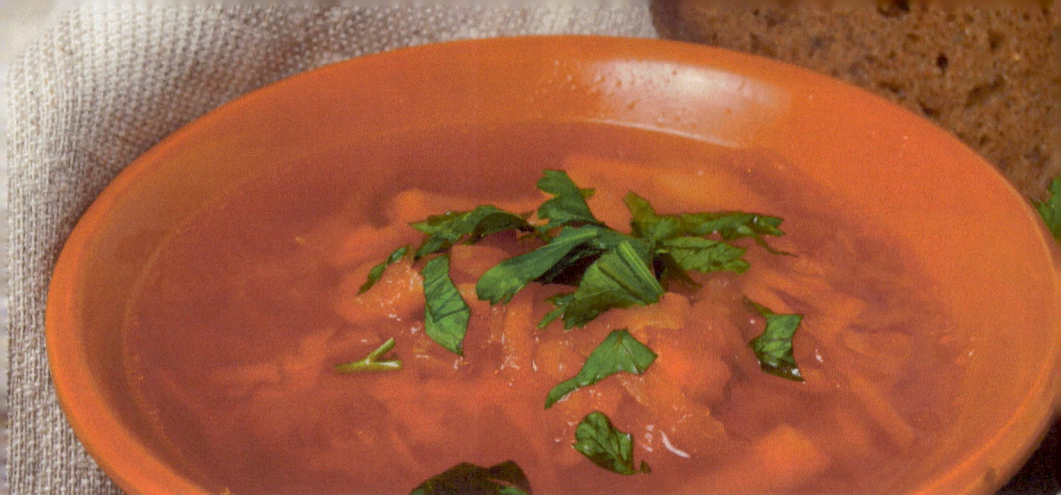

Beetroot and Cabbage Broth

500 ml water

50 g cabbage

1 sweet potato   1 beetroot

1 orange   Parsley

Bring 1 litre water to boil in a pan. Cut potato in the quarter. Chop cabbage and add to boiling water. Peel beetroots and grate. Add the next two beetroots in a juicer. Add orange to a juicer. Pour juice into the pan. Bring all ingredients to simmer. Add parsley for garnish.

FOOD	NUTRITIONAL BENEFITS
Cabbage	Fights inflammation, promotes a healthy gut, combats chronic disease
Beetroot	Good source of Iron and folate. Helps to lower blood pressure, boost exercise performance and prevent dementia
Sweet potato	Superfood. Good for diabetes. Anti-cancer. Immune system booster.
Orange	Anti-diabetes, skin food, heart healthy, anti-cancer, vitamin c rich
Red cabbage	Fights inflammation, promotes a healthy gut, combats chronic disease

Pineapple Pina Colada

5 cm slice of pineapple

1 fresh red or green chili (2cm)

1 peach or nectarine

Peel pineapple and cut in cubes. Remove stone from peach. Place all in a smoothie machine

FOOD	NUTRITIONAL BENEFITS
Pineapple	Eye health, enzyme rich, reduce allergies, ease digestion
Chili	Cleanse sinus, aids digestion, relieve migraine & muscle pain
Peach	Immune system booster, relief from cancer. Antioxidants. Skin health.
Nectarine	Protects against free radicals, skin and tendon health.

DAY 7

Are you feeling revitalised?
One week hooray – Congratulations!!!

Breakfast
Super Green Smoothie

Lunch
Lime and Rocket Herbal

Dinner
Coconut, Ginger and Pumpkin Soup

Extra Boost
Horseradish and Beetroot Blast

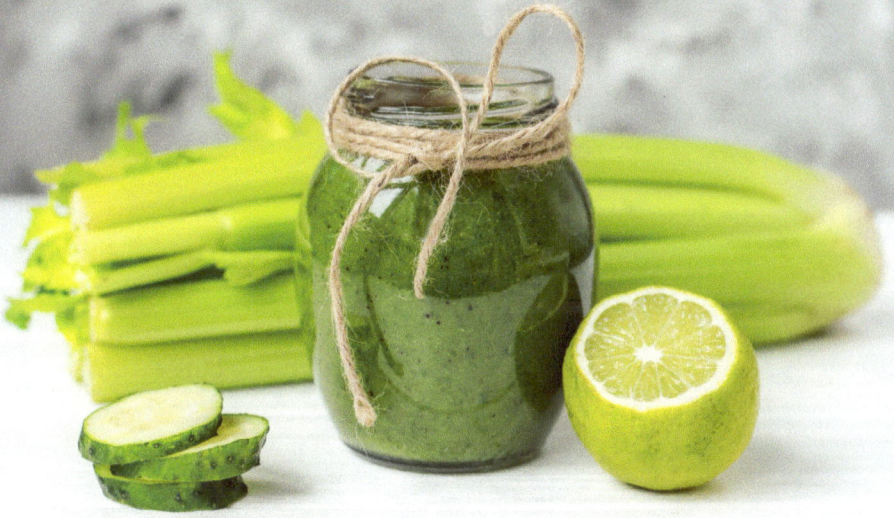

Super Green Smoothie

1 avocado

1 golden delicious apple

400ml coconut water

½ cucumber

1 handful spinach

5 stems parsley

5 stems mint

1 lime

1 cm root ginger

2 tablespoons hemp seed oil

3 stevia leaves

2 tablespoons flaxseed, pumpkin or olive oil

Juice spinach, parsley, mint, lime and root ginger. Pour mixture into a smoothie machine. Add coconut water, avocado, flaxseed, pumpkin seed and hemp seeds until smooth. Add stevia to taste.

FOOD	NUTRITIONAL BENEFITS
Avocado	Fiber-rich, heart healthy, brain healthy, good for the nervous system
Coconut water	Hydration. Electrolytes. Antioxidant.
Cucumber	Stress relief, hydration, skin health
Spinach	Superfood, nutrient-rich - skin, hair and bone health
Parsley	Good for kidney and bladder health. Cleanses & relieves constipation
Mint	Aids in digestion. Antiseptic, antibacterial, helps IBS & headaches
Lime	Cleanses blood, improves digestion and great for thyroid health.
Ginger	Powerful anti-inflammatory (good for arthritis), soothes the stomach
Flaxseed	Heart Healthy. Omega 2 rich. Lubricates joints.
Hemp seeds	Protein-rich, brain health, heart healthy, PMS support
Stevia	No calories, anti-cancer, good for diabetes.
Apple	Rich in antioxidants, flavonoids and dietary fibre. Helps hypertension, diabetes, cancer and heart disease

Lime and Rocket Zest

A handful of rocket leaves 1 lime

½ cucumber 1 teaspoon flaxseed or olive oil

4 celery stalks

Peel Lime, Juice celery stalks, lime, rocket leaves and cucumber. Add flaxseed and olive oil on top.

FOOD	NUTRITIONAL BENEFITS
Rocket	Rocket (aka. arugula) High in vitamin c. Powerful antioxidant
Cucumber	Stress relief, hydration, skin health
Celery	Rich in antioxidants and beneficial enzymes
Lime	Cleanses blood, improves digestion and great for thyroid health.
Flaxseed	Heart Healthy. Omega 2 rich. Lubricates joints.
Olive oil	Antioxidant-rich, anti-inflammatory, prevent strokes, heart healthy

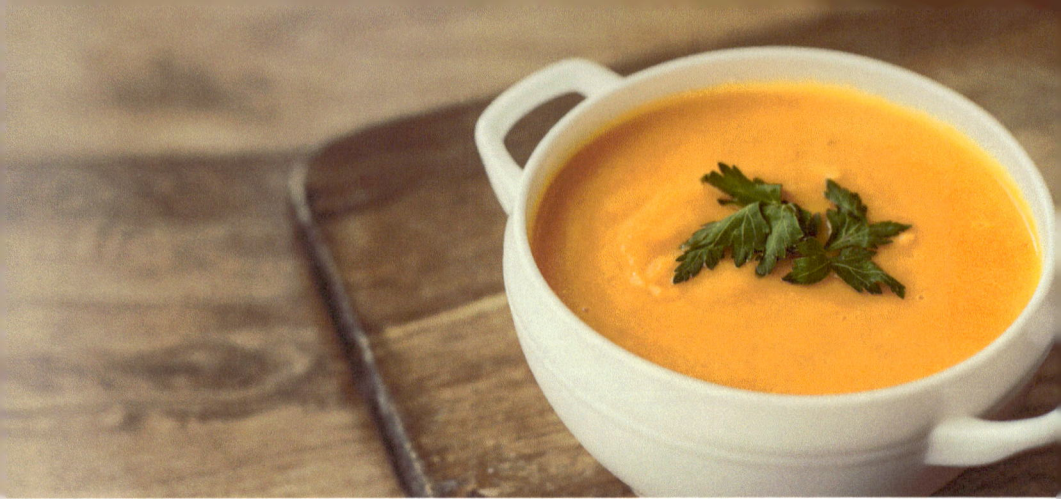

Coconut, Pumpkin and Ginger Soup

1 cm root ginger

1 tablespoon turmeric

¼ small pumpkin

400 ml full-fat coconut milk

1 lime

100 ml water

Few almonds to garnish

Handful of coriander

Bring to boil in the water, pumpkin, ginger and onions. Stir in the turmeric. Add coconut milk and stir. Simmer for 10 minutes. Pour mixture into a smoothie machine or blender until smooth. Add almonds and coriander to serve.

FOOD	NUTRITIONAL BENEFITS
Ginger	Powerful anti-inflammatory (good for arthritis), soothes the stomach
Turmeric	Healing benefits, anti-inflammatory, antioxidant.
Pumpkin	Fiber, potassium, and vitamin C. Helps high blood pressure
Coconut milk	Lowers Blood Pressure & Cholesterol. Helps Prevent Anaemia
Lime	Cleanses blood, improves digestion and great for thyroid health.
Almonds	Relieves Stress. May prevent cardiovascular disease.
Coriander	Cleansing, reduce infections, lower blood sugars

Horseradish and Beetroot Blast

125 ml water

1 lemon

1 cm horseradish

1 beetroot

Peel lemon. Cut lemon and beetroot in dices. Add to a juicer. Grate horseradish into the juice and mix well.

FOOD	NUTRITIONAL BENEFITS
Lemon	Anti-parasitic, alkalizing all round cleanser
Horseradish	Purify blood, cleanse liver and stomach.
Beetroot	Amazing for blood & liver health. Increases oxygen in blood.

DAY 8

Another week of more energising and tasty juice, smoothies and soups!

Breakfast
Berry Smoothie

Lunch
Broccoli Boost

Dinner
Coconut, ginger and Carrot Soup

Extra Boost
Pineapple and lemon shot

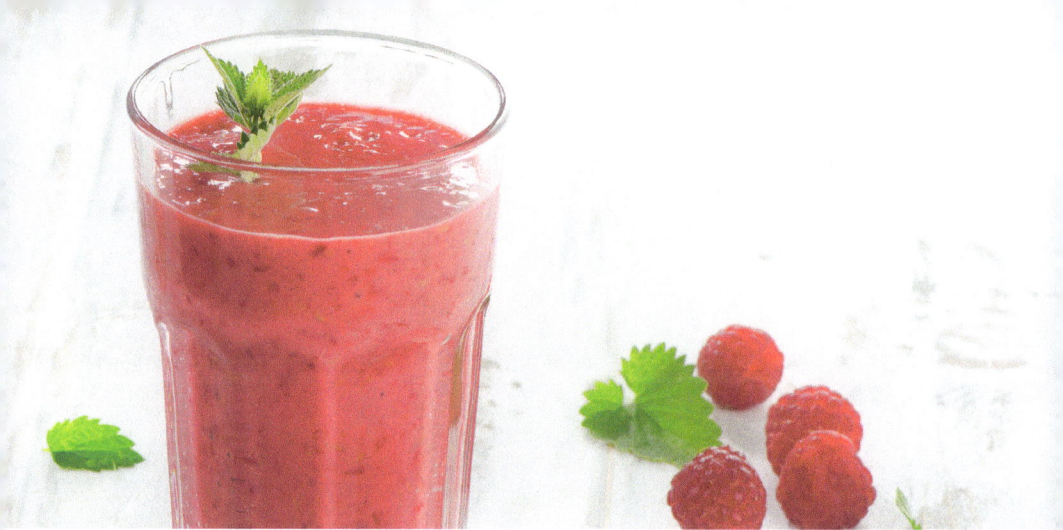

Berry Smoothie

1 teaspoon flaxseed

1 teaspoon pumpkin seeds

1 teaspoon sunflower seeds

1 cup fresh berries (blueberries, strawberries)

1 small banana

½ lemon

350 ml coconut water

Wash produce. Peel banana and lemon. Place all ingredients in a blender. Puree all ingredients using a smoothie machine or blender until smooth.

FOOD	NUTRITIONAL BENEFITS
Flaxseed	Heart Healthy. Omega 2 rich. Lubricates joints.
Pumpkin seeds	Nutritional powerhouse, good for nerves, anti-oxidant, protein rich
Sunflower seeds	Heart healthy, antioxidant, good for thyroid health and mood.
Banana	Fibre rich, ease digestion, prevent anaemia
Blueberries	Heart Health, fibre rich, clean blood
Strawberries	Overall health, rich in vitamins, fibre, minerals.
Lemon	Anti-parasitic, alkalizing all round cleanser
Coconut Water	Hydration. Electrolytes. Antioxidant.

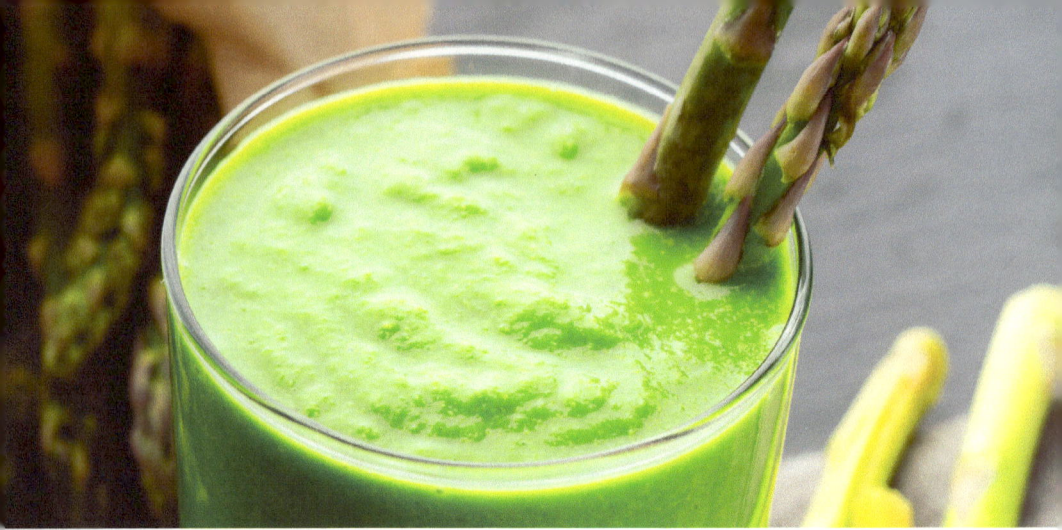

Broccoli Boost

3 stem broccoli	2 asparagus
1 celery stalk	1 medium parsnip
½ medium cucumber	2 apples (gala)

Wash all produce. Core apples, Juice all vegetables and fruits in a juicer- pour.

FOOD	NUTRITIONAL BENEFITS
Broccoli	Builds collagen - forms tissue and bone. Antioxidant.
Celery	Rich in antioxidants and beneficial enzymes
Cucumber	Stress relief, hydration, skin health
Asparagus	Helps fight cancer, good for cleansing the blood, rich in fiber, diuretic
Parsnip	High in potassium: Reduce blood pressure. Improve heart health.
Gala Apples	Cleanse colon, regulate blood sugar, lower cholesterol

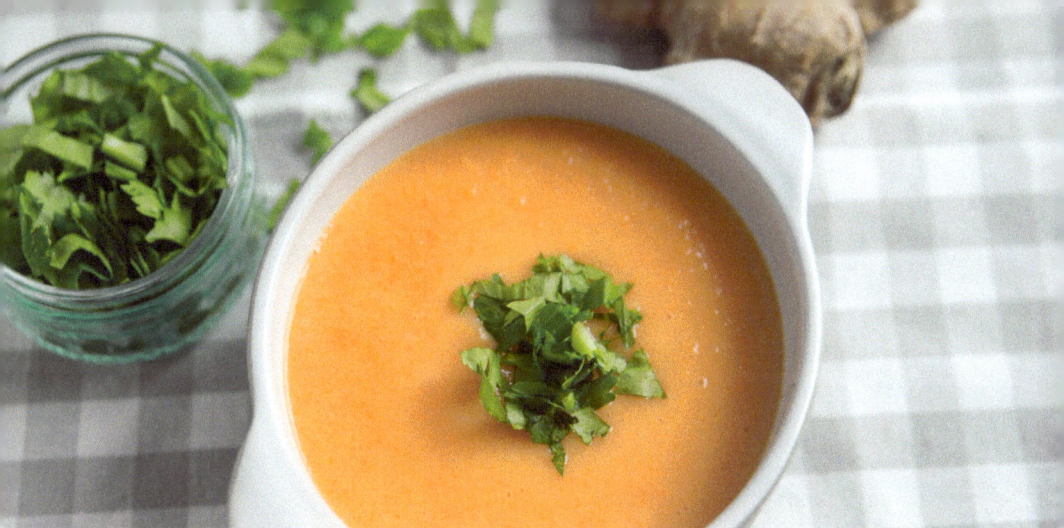

Coconut, Carrot and Ginger Soup

1 cm root ginger

1 tablespoon turmeric

200 g carrots

400 ml full-fat coconut milk

1 lime

750 ml water

Few almonds to garnish

Handful of coriander

Bring to boil in the water, carrots, ginger and onions. Stir in the turmeric. Add coconut milk and stir. Simmer for 10 minutes. Leave to cool and then pour mixture into a smoothie machine or blender until smooth. Add almonds and coriander to serve.

FOOD	NUTRITIONAL BENEFITS
Ginger	Powerful anti-inflammatory (good for arthritis), soothes the stomach
Turmeric	Healing benefits, anti-inflammatory, antioxidant.
Carrots	Rich in beta-carotene: for healthy skin, immune system & eye health
Coconut Milk	Lowers Blood Pressure & Cholesterol. Helps Prevent Anaemia
Lime	Cleanses blood, improves digestion and great for thyroid health.
Almonds	Relieves Stress. May prevent cardiovascular disease.
Coriander	Cleansing, reduce infections, lower blood sugars

Pineapple and Lemon Shot

¼ pineapple

1 lemon

1 stalk mint

Peel pineapple and lemon. Wash mint. Juice pineapple and lemon. Add mint as a garnish on top.

FOOD	NUTRITIONAL BENEFITS
Pineapple	Eye health, enzyme rich, reduce allergies, ease digestion
Lemon	Anti-parasitic, alkalizing all round cleanser
Mint	Aids in digestion. Antiseptic, antibacterial, helps IBS & headaches

DAY 9

Breakfast
Beetroot, Carrots and Celery Powerhouse

Lunch
Spinach, Pear and Lime Juice

Dinner
Vegetable Tea

Extra Boost
Cherry Tonic

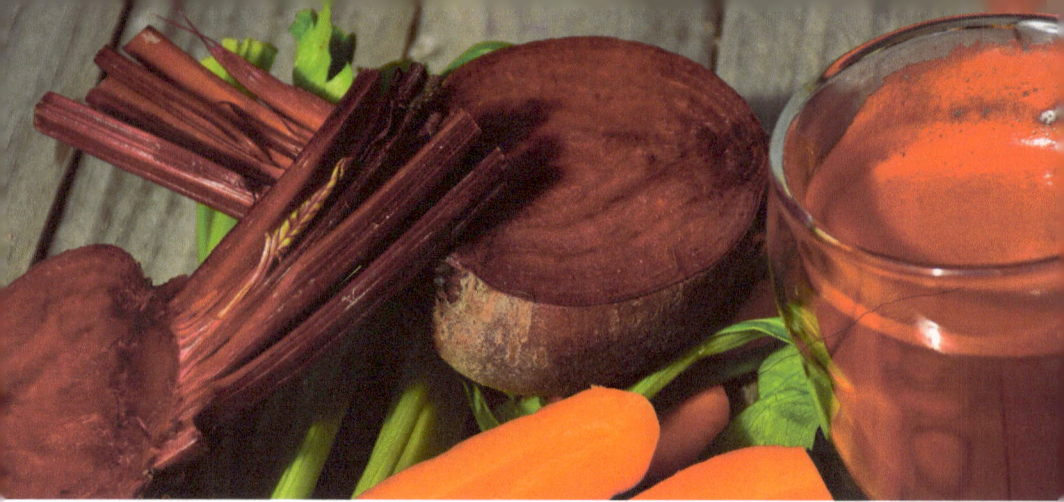

Beetroot, Carrots & Celery Powerhouse

1 raw beetroot, chopped

1 large carrot, chopped

2 stalks celery

2 green apples

1 teaspoon pumpkin seeds

1 teaspoon avocado oil

Wash produce, core apples. Juice beetroot, carrot, celery and green apples. Add pumpkin seeds and avocado oil on top.

FOOD	NUTRITIONAL BENEFITS
Beetroot	Amazing for blood & liver health. Increases oxygen in blood.
Carrot	Rich in beta carotene: for healthy skin, immune system & eye health
Celery	Rich in antioxidants and beneficial enzymes
Apples	Cleanse colon, regulate blood sugar, lower cholesterol
Pumpkin seeds	Nutritional powerhouse, good for nerves, anti-oxidant, protein-rich
Avocado oil	Heart-healthy, brain healthy, good for the nervous system

Spinach, Pear and Lime Juice

1 small handful spinach

1 green apple

1 conference pear

Lime, unwaxed

½ cucumber

1 celery stalk

Juice all vegetables and fruits in a juicer

Wash produce. Core apple. Peel lime. Place greens in a juicer and then the rest – juice and pour.

FOOD	NUTRITIONAL BENEFITS
Spinach	Super food, nutrient-rich - skin, hair and bone health
Apple	Cleanse colon, regulate blood sugar, lower cholesterol
Pear	Calms nerves, supple joints, and good for gout/arthritis. Mild laxative.
Lime	Cleanses blood, improves digestion and great for thyroid health.
Cucumber	Stress relief, hydration, skin health
Celery	Rich in antioxidants and beneficial enzymes

Vegetable Tea

1 celery stalk, chopped   Coriander stalk

1 carrot, chopped   2 bay leaves

1 sweet potato, chopped   1 tablespoon chopped lovage

½ fennel bulb, chopped   Himalayan salt

Parsley stalk

Peel and chop sweet potato, carrots, lovage, celery and fennel. Add vegetables to boiling water, leave to simmer for 20 minutes. Add bay leaves and coriander to water for another 5 minutes. Add Himalayan salt to taste.

FOOD	NUTRITIONAL BENEFITS
Celery	Rich in antioxidants and beneficial enzymes
Carrot	Rich in beta carotene: for healthy skin, immune system & eye health
Sweet potato	Super food. Good for diabetes. Anti-cancer. Immune system booster.
Fennel	Cleansing benefits, rich in vitamin B6, antioxidant rich, calcium rich
Parsley	Good for kidney and bladder health. Cleanses & relieves constipation
Coriander	Cleansing, reduce infections, lower blood sugars
Bay leaves	Ease joint pain, muscle relief, good for arthritis, nutrient rich.
Himalayan salt	Balance pH and blood sugar. Detoxify body. Improves hydration.

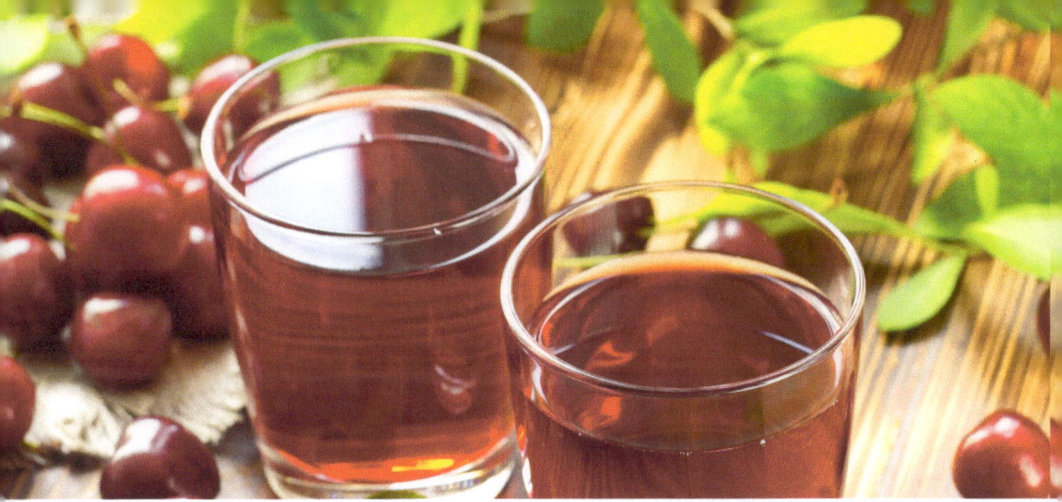

Cherry Tonic

15 cherries

250 ml coconut water

Remove seeds from cherries. Pour 100ml coconut water and add cherries to smoothie machine. Blend until smooth. Enjoy!

FOOD	NUTRITIONAL BENEFITS
Cherry	Reduce belly fat, promote healthy sleep, antioxidant rich, reduce muscle pain
Coconut water	Hydration. Electrolytes. Antioxidant.

DAY 10

Breakfast
Grapefruit Punch

Lunch
Super Green Smoothie

Dinner
Vegetables, Spinach & Okra Soup

Extra Boost
Celery and Cucumber Blast

Grapefruit Punch

1 lime, peeled   4 satsumas, peeled

2 peeled oranges   1 pink grapefruit, peeled

Peel Grapefruit, satsumas and lime. Puree all ingredients using a smoothie machine or blender.

FOOD	NUTRITIONAL BENEFITS
Grapefruit	Maintain a healthy heart and blood pressure
Lime	Cleanses blood, improves digestion and great for thyroid health.
Nutmeg	Great all round detoxifier, skin health, releive pain
Satsuma	Good source of vitamin A, B1, B2, B3, B5, B6, B9 (Folate), C and E and calcium, iron, magnesium, manganese, phosphorus, potassium, zinc and dietary fibre.

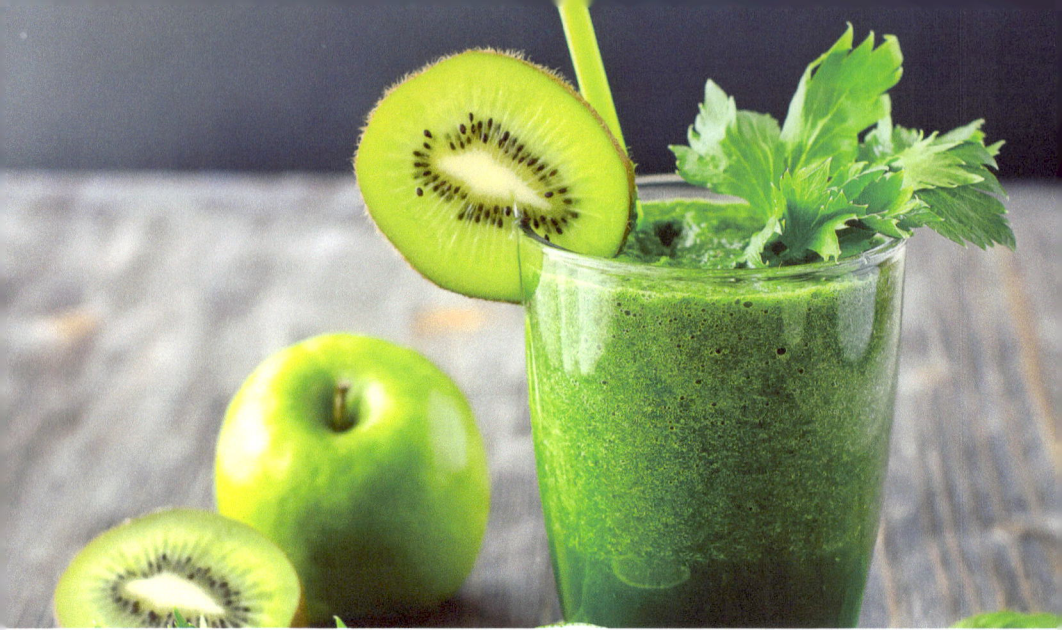

Super Green Kiwi Smoothie

2 small kiwi

1 large handful kale

1 large handful spinach

2 medium green apples

½ unwaxed lime

2 broccoli stem

1 small avocado

1 heaped teaspoon spirulina

1 teaspoon wheatgrass

Juice all vegetables and fruits in a juicer. Transfer to a smoothie machine, add avocado (without seed), spirulina and wheatgrass. Mix until smooth

FOOD	NUTRITIONAL BENEFITS
Avocado	Fibre-rich, heart healthy, brain healthy, good for the nervous system
Coconut Water	Hydration. Electrolytes. Antioxidant.
Cucumber	Stress relief, hydration, skin health
Spinach	Superfood, nutrient-rich - skin, hair and bone health
Parsley	Good for kidney and bladder health. Cleanses & relieves constipation
Mint	Aids in digestion. Antiseptic, antibacterial, helps IBS & headaches
Lime	Cleanses blood, improves digestion and great for thyroid health.
Ginger	Powerful anti-inflammatory (good for arthritis), soothes the stomach
Flaxseed	Heart Healthy. Omega 2 rich. Lubricates joints.
Hemp seeds	Protein-rich, brain health, heart healthy, PMS support
Stevia	No calories, anti-cancer, good for diabetes.
Kiwi	Super food with over 20 nutrients. Skin health. Reduce blood pressure

Vegetables, Spinach & Okra Soup

Vegetable tea (day nine)   1 stalk coriander

1 handful spinach   Himalayan salt

1 stalk parsley   6 okra

To the vegetable tea, add spinach, okra, parsley and coriander for 10 minutes. Add Himalayan salt to taste.

FOOD	NUTRITIONAL BENEFITS
Spinach	Superfood, nutrient-rich - skin, hair and bone health
Parsley	Good for kidney and bladder health. Cleanses & relieves constipation
Coriander	Cleansing, reduce infections, lower blood sugars
Himalayan salt	Balance pH and blood sugar. Detoxify body. Improves hydration.
Okra	Rich in potassium, vitamin B, vitamin C, folic acid, and calcium. It's low in calories and has a high dietary fibre content.

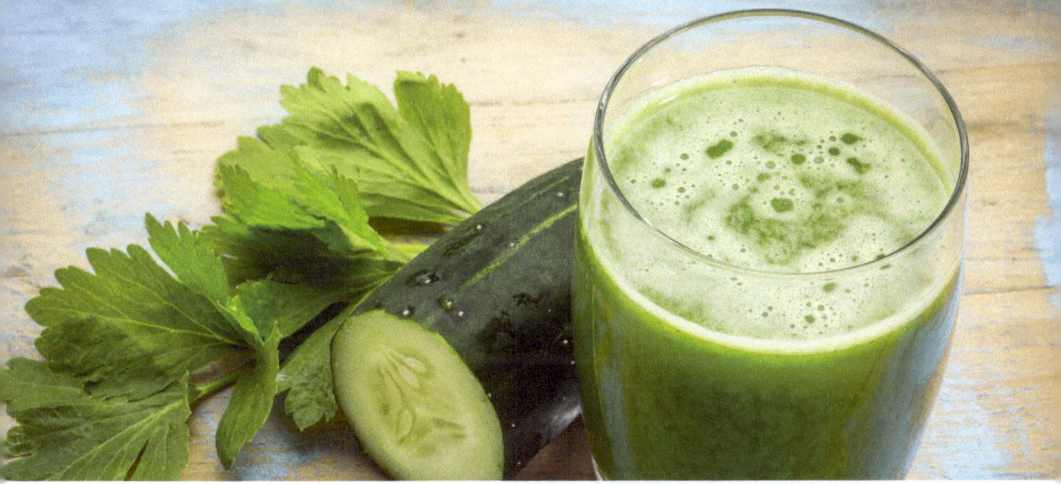

Celery & Cucumber Blast

½ lemon

2 celery stalks

½ cucumber

Wash produce. Juice cucumber and celery together.

FOOD	NUTRITIONAL BENEFITS
Celery	Rich in antioxidants and beneficial enzymes
Cucumber	Stress relief, hydration, skin health

DAY 11

Breakfast
Beetroot, Carrots and Celery Juice

Lunch
Spinach, Pear and Lime Juice

Dinner
Leek and Coriander Cream Soup

Extra Boost
Cherry Tonic

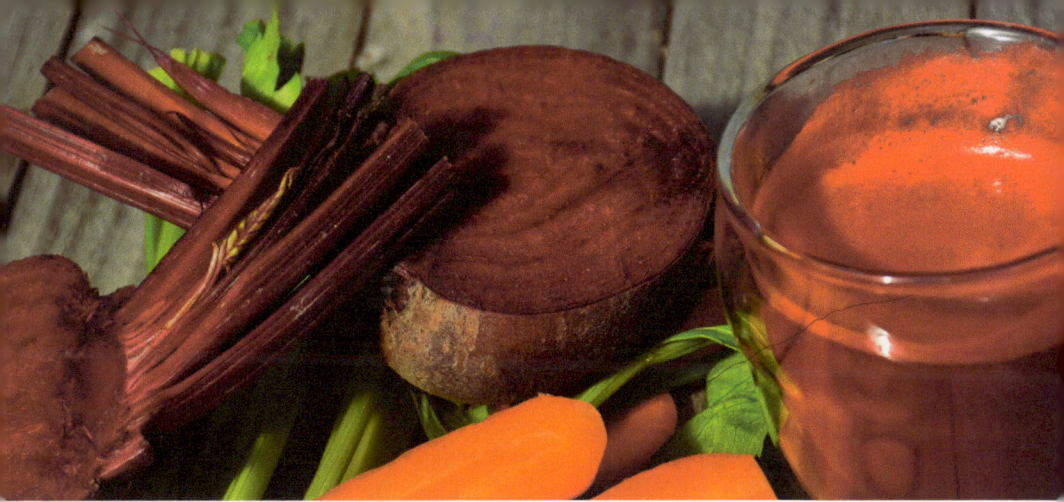

Beetroot, Carrots & Celery Juice

1 raw beetroot, chopped

1 large carrot, chopped

2 stalks celery

2 green apples

1 teaspoon pumpkin seeds

1 teaspoon avocado oil

Wash produce. Core apples. Juice beetroot, carrot, celery and green apples. Add pumpkin seeds and avocado oil on top.

FOOD	NUTRITIONAL BENEFITS
Beetroot	Amazing for blood & liver health. Increases oxygen in the blood.
Carrot	Rich in beta-carotene: for healthy skin, immune system & eye health
Celery	Rich in antioxidants and beneficial enzymes
Apples	Cleanse colon, regulate blood sugar, lower cholesterol
Pumpkin seeds	A nutritional powerhouse, good for nerves, anti-oxidant, protein-rich
Avocado oil	Heart-healthy, brain healthy, good for the nervous system

Spinach, Pear and Lime Juice

1 small handful spinach

1 green apple

1 conference pear

Lime, unwaxed

½ cucumber

1 celery stalk

Wash produce. Core apple. Peel lime. Juice all vegetables and fruits in a juicer, starting with the spinach.

FOOD	NUTRITIONAL BENEFITS
Spinach	Super food, nutrient-rich - skin, hair and bone health
Apple	Cleanse colon, regulate blood sugar, lower cholesterol
Pear	Calms nerves, supple joints, and good for gout/arthritis. Mild laxative.
Lime	Cleanses blood, improves digestion and great for thyroid health.
Cucumber	Stress relief, hydration, skin health
Celery	Rich in antioxidants and beneficial enzymes

Leek and Coriander Cream Soup

2 leeks

2 stalks coriander   1 onion

1 handful spinach   Himalayan salt

1 stalk parsley   1 small sweet potato

2 parsnips   750 ml water

Bring to boil water. Wash vegetables. Add spinach, chopped onions, sweet potato, leek, and parsnips. Bring to boil for 15 minutes. Add chopped parsley, coriander and Himalayan salt.

FOOD	NUTRITIONAL BENEFITS
Spinach	Superfood, nutrient-rich - skin, hair and bone health
Parsley	Good for kidney and bladder health. Cleanses & relieves constipation
Coriander	Cleansing, reduce infections, lower blood sugars
Himalayan salt	Balance pH and blood sugar. Detoxify body. Improves hydration.
Leek	Good source of vitamin A, E, K, manganese, vitamin B6, copper, calcium, omega 3 fatty acid, magnesium, iron, folate and vitamin C.
Parsnip	High levels of minerals: calcium, potassium, manganese, magnesium, phosphorous, zinc, and iron. Good source of fibre, folate, thiamin, pantothenic acid, vitamin B6, C, E, and K

Cherry Tonic

15 cherries

250 ml coconut water

Remove seeds from cherries. Pour 100ml coconut water and add cherries to smoothie machine. Blend until smooth.

FOOD	NUTRITIONAL BENEFITS
Cherry	Reduce belly fat, promote healthy sleep, antioxidant rich, reduce muscle pain
Coconut Water	Hydration. Electrolytes. Antioxidant.

DAY 12

Breakfast
Cucumber and Watermelon Chiller

Lunch
Red Pepper Juice

Dinner
Sweet Potato Smoothie

Extra Boost
Kale Espresso

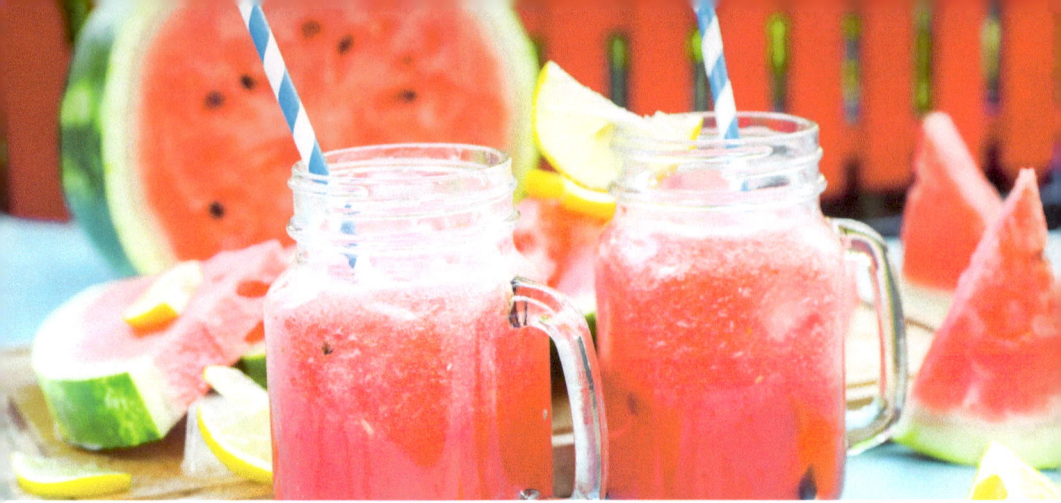

Cucumber & Watermelon Chiller

2 large slices of watermelon

1 cucumber, chunks

2 limes

Peel lime. Dice watermelon. Juice cucumber, watermelon and limes in a juicer.

FOOD	NUTRITIONAL BENEFITS
Watermelon	Increase blood flow. Immune System Support.
Cucumber	Stress relief, hydration, skin health
Lime	Cleanses blood, improves digestion and great for thyroid health.

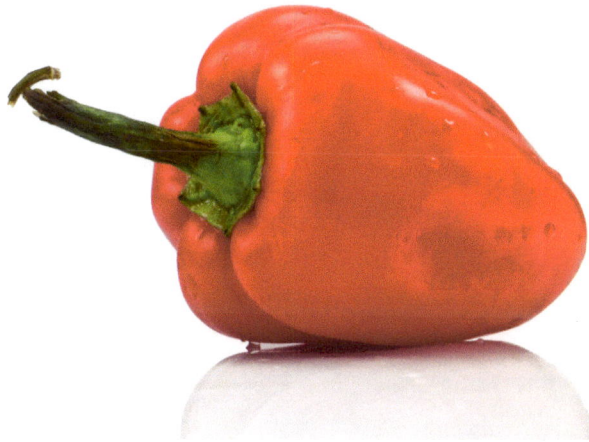

Red Pepper Juice

1 handful of spinach

1 red pepper

1 bunch red grapes

1 green or red apple

Wash produce. Core apple. Remove stem and pips from the pepper. Juice all vegetables and fruits in a juicer.

FOOD	NUTRITIONAL BENEFITS
Spinach	Superfood, nutrient-rich - skin, hair and bone health
Pepper	Anti-inflammatory, multiple health benefits. Protects against cancer.
Grapes	Fights cancer, constipation relief, anti-diabetic, relief from allergies
Apple	Cleanse colon, regulate blood sugar, lower cholesterol

Sweet Potato Smoothie

1 lemon

2 carrots   2 oranges

1 small sweet potato   500 ml water

Peel potatoes and cut into chunks. Place carrots, oranges and sweet potato in a smoothie machine.

FOOD	NUTRITIONAL BENEFITS
Carrot	Rich in beta-carotene: for healthy skin, immune system & eye health
Sweet Potato	Superfood. Good for diabetes. Anti-cancer. Immune system booster.
Oranges	Anti-diabetes, skin food, heart healthy, anti-cancer, vitamin c rich
Lemon	Anti-parasitic, alkalizing all round cleanser

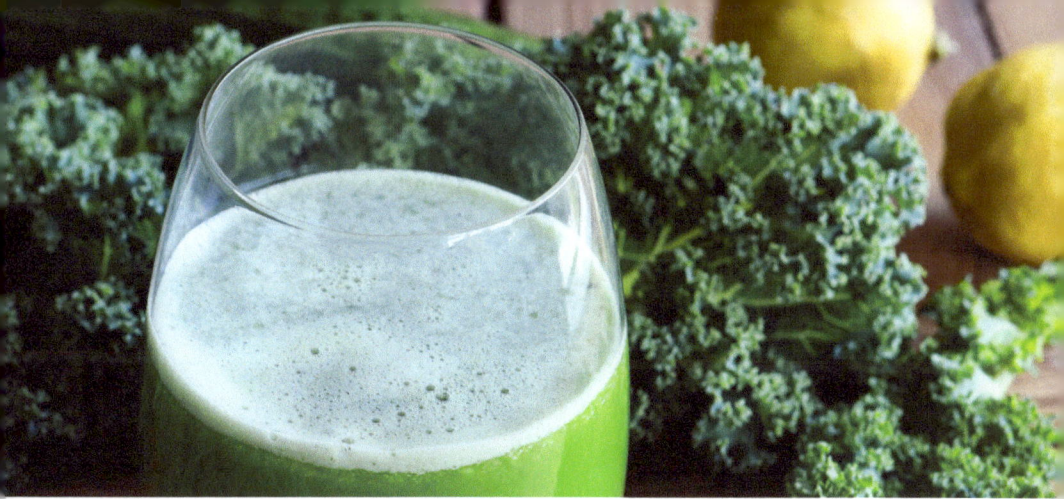

Kale Espresso

1 unwaxed lemon

1 green apple, peeled

1 handful of kale

2 cm root ginger

1 stalk of mint

Add unwaxed lemon, peeled green apple, kale and root ginger to the juicer. Transfer to a glass, add mint and stir.

FOOD	NUTRITIONAL BENEFITS
Lemon	Anti-parasitic, alkalizing all round cleanser
Apple	Cleanse colon, regulate blood sugar, lower cholesterol
Kale	High in iron, zero fat, prevent cancer, anti-inflammatory
Ginger	Powerful anti-inflammatory (good for arthritis), soothes the stomach
Mint	Aids in digestion. Antiseptic, antibacterial, helps IBS & headaches

DAY 13

Breakfast
Pineapple & Kiwi Cooler

Lunch
Fennel, Courgette and Pear Juice

Dinner
Cabbage Soup

Extra Boost
Mango Crush

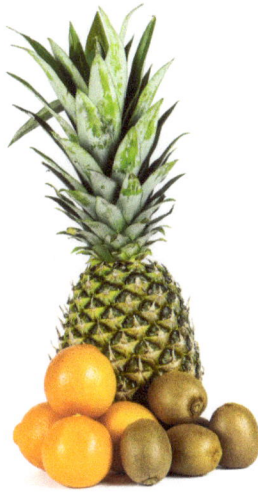

Pineapple & Kiwi Cooler

½ pineapple

1 kiwi

1 lime

mint leaves

Peel and dice pineapple. Peel kiwi and lime. Juice all vegetables and fruits in a juicer.

FOOD	NUTRITIONAL BENEFITS
Pineapple	Eye health, enzyme rich, reduce allergies, ease digestion
Kiwi	Super food with over 20 nutrients. Skin health. Reduce blood pressure
Lime	Cleanses blood, improves digestion and great for thyroid health.
Mint	Aids in digestion. Antiseptic, antibacterial, helps IBS & headaches

Fennel, Courgette & Pear Juice

2 pears

1 courgette

¼ fennel

3 stem broccoli

1 handful of spinach

Wash produce. Cut pears, courgette and fennel in chunks. Place in a juicer adding broccoli, but juice spinach first.

FOOD	NUTRITIONAL BENEFITS
Pears	Calms nerves, supple joints, and good for gout/arthritis. Mild laxative.
Courgette	Control diabetes, eye healthy, improves digestion. Anti-inflammatory.
Fennel	Cleansing benefits, rich in vitamin B6, antioxidant-rich, calcium-rich
Broccoli	Builds collagen - forms tissue and bone. Antioxidant.
Spinach	Super food, nutrient-rich - skin, hair and bone health

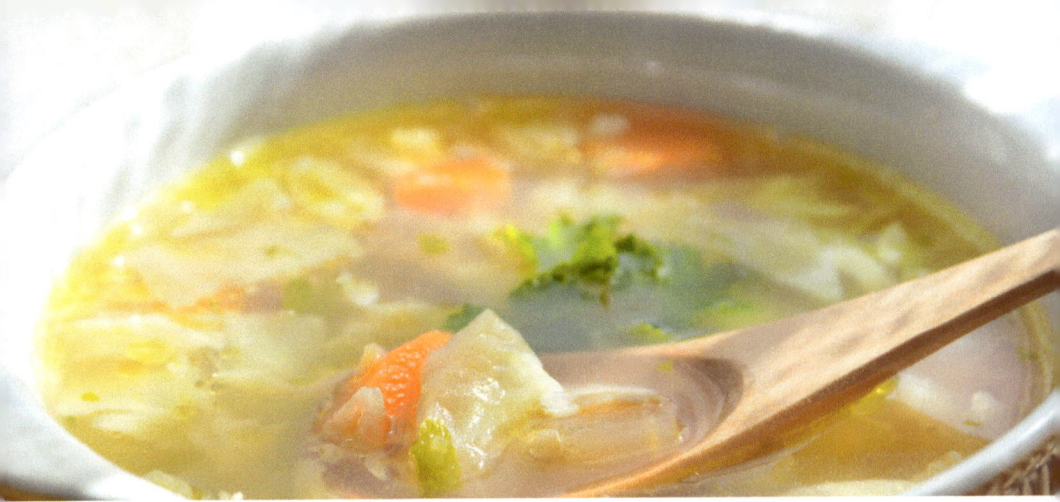

Cabbage Soup

1 green pepper

1 carrot

2 stalks celery

½ white cabbage

2 stalks parsley

½ red chili

Himalayan salt

1 litre water

Cut green pepper, carrots, celery and cabbage in chunks. Add water and bring to simmer for 20 minutes. Add Himalayan salt to taste.

FOOD	NUTRITIONAL BENEFITS
Green pepper	Anti-inflammatory, multiple health benefits. Protects against cancer.
Carrot	Rich in beta-carotene: for healthy skin, immune system & eye health
Celery	Rich in antioxidants and beneficial enzymes
Cabbage	Fights inflammation, promotes a healthy gut, combats chronic disease
Parsley	Good for kidney and bladder health. Cleanses & relieves constipation
Chilli	Cleanse sinus, aids digestion, relieve migraine & muscle pain
Himalayan salt	Balance pH and blood sugar. Detoxify body. Improves hydration.

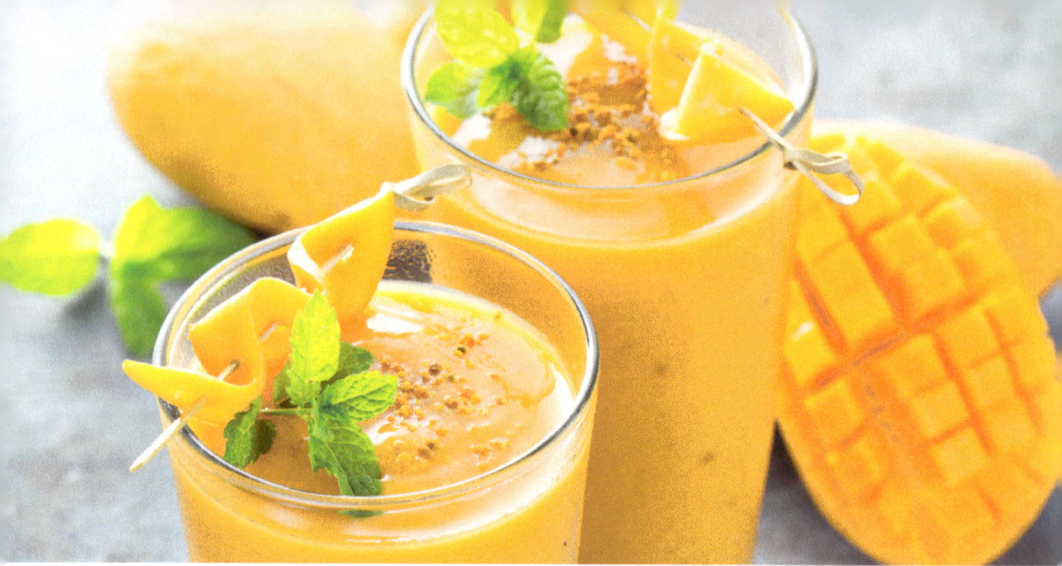

Mango Crush

1 mango

1 stalk mint

375 ml water

½ unwaxed lemon

Peel lemon and mango. Cut lemon and mango in chunks. Add to a smoothie machine. Blend until smooth, then add mint.

FOOD	NUTRITIONAL BENEFITS
Lemon	Anti-parasitic, alkalizing all round cleanser
Mango	Skin and eye health. Helps fight cancer. Improves digestion
Mint	Aids in digestion. Antiseptic, antibacterial, helps IBS & headaches

DAY 14

Breakfast
Beetroot and Ginger Juice

Lunch
Berries & Lettuce Smoothie

Dinner
Cabbage & Spinach Soup

Extra Boost
Passion Fruit and Apple Chiller

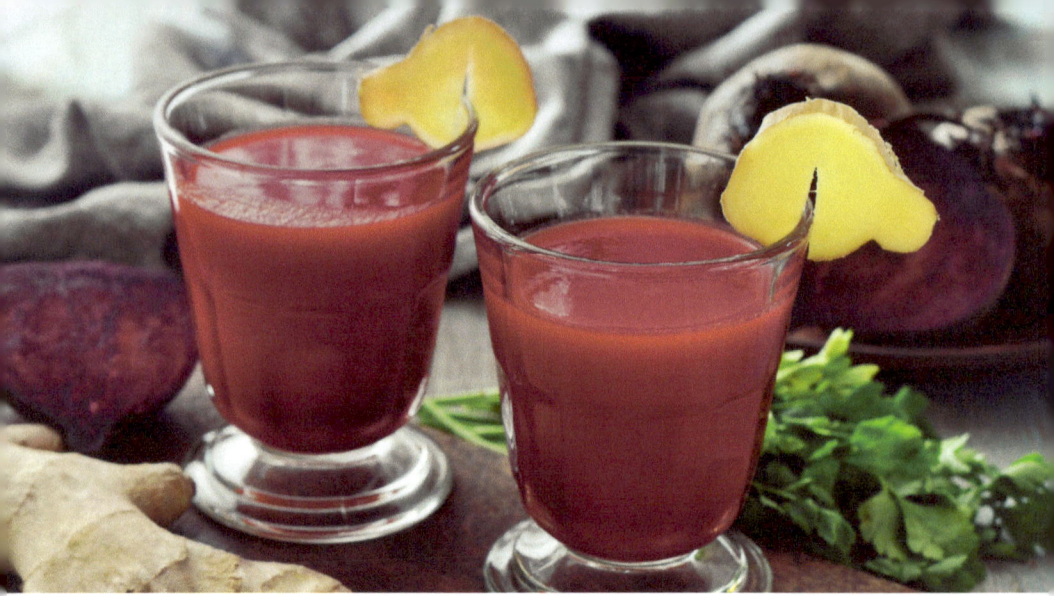

Beetroot and Ginger Juice

2 carrots

2 celery stalks

2 cm root ginger

1 beetroot

1 parsnip

1 apple

½ tablespoon pumpkin seed

Parsley

Avocado oil

Core apple. Chop vegetables and fruits to size to fit in your juicer. Juice all vegetables and fruits in a juicer. Add pumpkin seed, parsley and avocado oil and mix well.

FOOD	NUTRITIONAL BENEFITS
Celery	Rich in antioxidants and beneficial enzymes
Ginger	Powerful anti-inflammatory (good for arthritis), soothes stomach
Beetroot	Amazing for blood & liver health. Increases oxygen in blood.
Parsnip	High in potassium: Reduce blood pressure. Improve heart health.
Carrots	Rich in beta carotene: for healthy skin, immune system & eye health
Apple	Cleanse colon, regulate blood sugar, lower cholesterol
Pumpkin Seed	Nutritional powerhouse, good for nerves, antioxidant, protein rich
Parsley	Good for kidney and bladder health. Cleanses & relieves constipation
Avocado Oil	Heart & brain healthy, good for nervous system

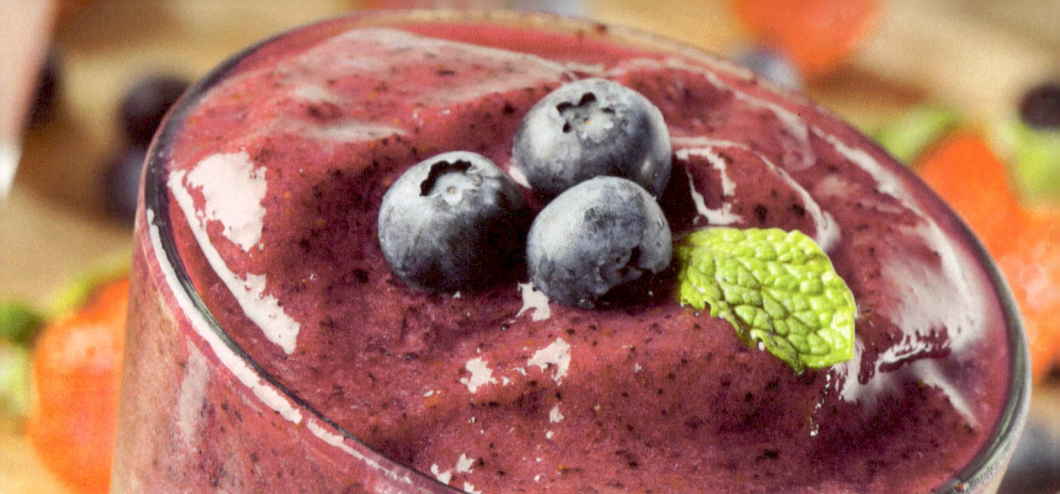

Berries and Lettuce Smoothie

½ cucumber

4 romaine lettuce

2 celery stalks

25 g blue berries

25 g strawberries

25 raspberries

375 ml water

Juice cucumber, lettuce and celery in a juicer. Transfer to a smoothie machine, add water and berries. Mixed until smooth.

FOOD	NUTRITIONAL BENEFITS
Cucumber	Stress relief, hydration, skin health
Romaine	Fight free radicals, bone strength, eye health
Celery	Rich in antioxidants and beneficial enzymes
Blueberries	Heart Health, fibre rich, clean blood
Strawberries	Overall health, rich in vitamins, fibre, minerals.
Raspberries	Antioxidant-rich, fight cancer, anti-aging

Cabbage & Spinach Soup

Cabbage soup (Day Thirteen)   6 Peppercorns

1 handful spinach   Himalayan salt

Coriander

Add spinach, peppercorn and coriander to cabbage soup from day thirteen. Bring to simmer for 10 minutes. Add Himalayan salt to taste.

FOOD	NUTRITIONAL BENEFITS
Cabbage	Fights inflammation, promotes a healthy gut, combats chronic disease
Spinach	Superfood, nutrient-rich - skin, hair and bone health
Coriander	Cleansing, reduce infections, lower blood sugars
Peppercorn	Helps transport nutrients, skin healthy, antioxidant, good for digestion
Himalayan salt	Balance pH and blood sugar. Detoxify body. Improves hydration.

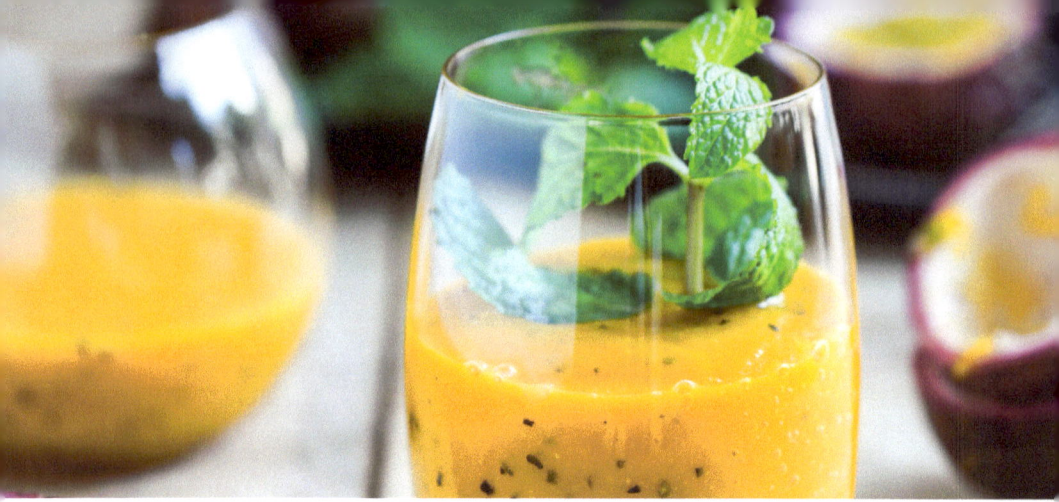

Passion Fruit Chiller

3 passion fruits

1 green apple

1 stalk mint

250 ml water

1 unwaxed lime

Core apple. Peel lime. Cut lime, apple and passion in chunks. Add to a smoothie machine. Blend until smooth, then add mint.

FOOD	NUTRITIONAL BENEFITS
Lime	Cleanses blood, improves digestion and great for thyroid health.
Passion fruit	Immune system booster, aids digestion, anti-cancer, improves circulation
Apple	Cleanse colon, regulate blood sugar, lower cholesterol
Mint	Aids in digestion. Antiseptic, antibacterial, helps IBS & headaches

DAY 15

Breakfast
Apple, Carrot & Parsley Juice

Lunch
Avocado & Kiwi Smoothie

Dinner
Butternut Squash & Ginger Soup

Extra Boost
Mango Crush

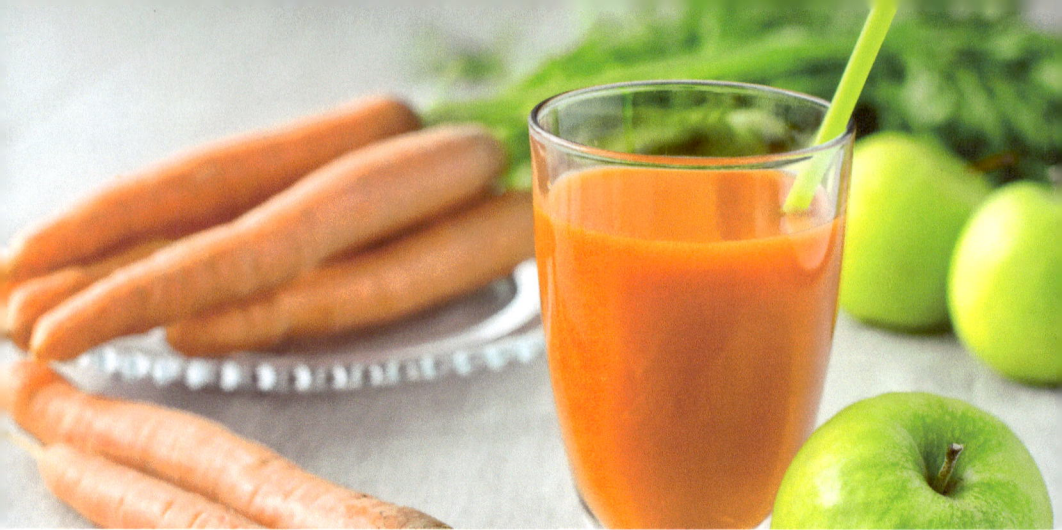

Apple, Carrot & Parsley Juice

2 green apple

2 large carrots

handful parsley

Wash produce. Core apple. Cut produce to size. Juice all vegetables and fruits in a juicer.

FOOD	NUTRITIONAL BENEFITS
Apple	Cleanse colon, regulate blood sugar, lower cholesterol
Carrots	Rich in beta-carotene: for healthy skin, immune system & eye health
Parsley	Good for kidney and bladder health. Cleanses & relieves constipation

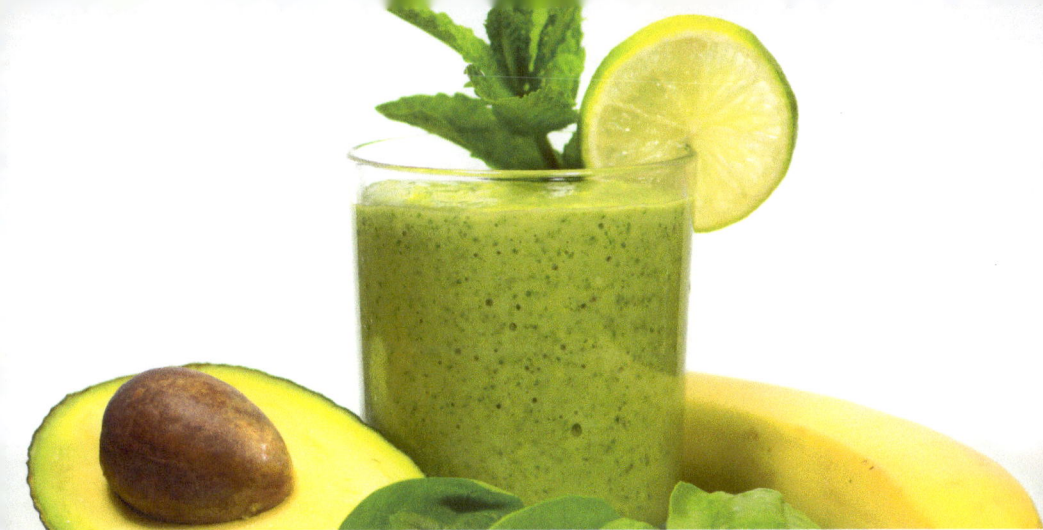

Avocado & Kiwi Smoothie

1 banana   2 limes

1 avocado   Handful of watercress

2 kiwi fruit   375 ml coconut water

Peel banana, avocado, limes and kiwi fruit. Remove avocado seed.
Put all ingredients in a smoothie machine with coconut water and
blend. Add watercress until smooth.

FOOD	NUTRITIONAL BENEFITS
Banana	Fibre rich, ease digestion, prevent anaemia
Avocado	Fibre-rich, heart healthy, brain healthy, good for the nervous system
Kiwi	Super food with over 20 nutrients. Skin health. Reduce blood pressure
Lime	Cleanses blood, improves digestion and great for thyroid health.
Watercress	Protects against cancer, antioxidant, bone & teeth strength.
Coconut water	Hydration. Electrolytes. Antioxidant.

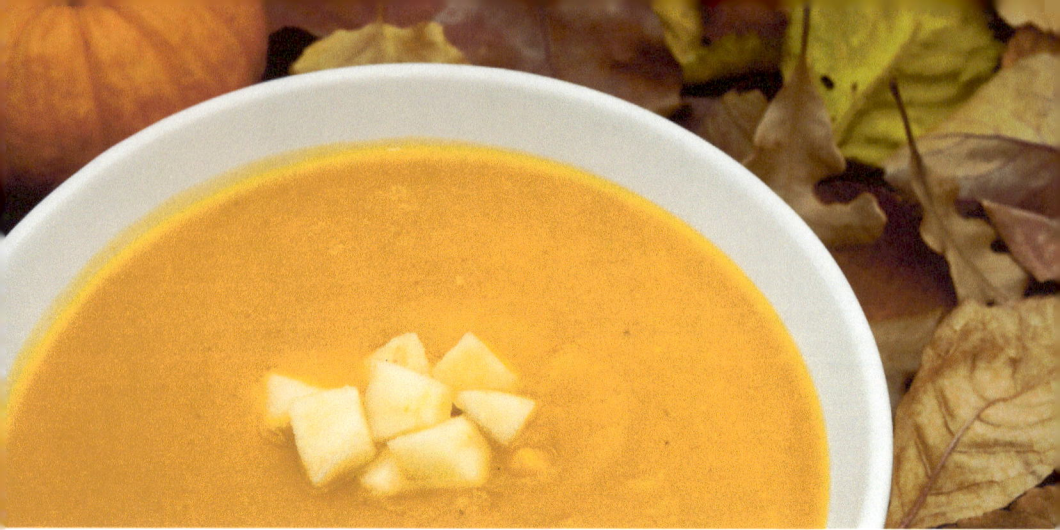

Butternut, Apple & Ginger Soup

2 butternut squash (peeled)   ½ green Apple

2 cm root ginger   Coriander

1 celery   Himalayan salt

1 leek   1 litre water

Wash produce. Chop leek, celery. Peel and chop butternut squash and ginger. Add butternut squash, root ginger, chopped celery and leek to water. Boil for 20 minutes. Add coriander and salt to taste. Pour mixture into a smoothie machine until smooth. Add chopped apple to garnish.

FOOD	NUTRITIONAL BENEFITS
Butternut squash	Good for bones, eyesight, skin and relieves constipation
Ginger	Powerful anti-inflammatory (good for arthritis), soothes the stomach
Celery	Rich in antioxidants and beneficial enzymes
Leek	Fight free radicals in your body. Anti-cancer. Anti-diabetes.
Coriander	Cleansing, reduce infections, lower blood sugars
Himalayan salt	Balance pH and blood sugar. Detoxify body. Improves hydration.

Mango Crush

1 mango

1 green apple

1 stalk mint

1 unwaxed lemon

375 ml water

Peel lemon and mango. Cut lemon apple and mango in chunks. Add to a smoothie machine. Blend until smooth, then add mint.

FOOD	NUTRITIONAL BENEFITS
Lemon	Anti-parasitic, alkalizing all round cleanser
Mango	Skin and eye health. Helps fight cancer. Improves digestion
Mint	Aids in digestion. Antiseptic, antibacterial, helps IBS & headaches

DAY 16

Breakfast
Broccoli Power Juice

Lunch
Spinach Energy Smoothie

Dinner
Butternut Squash, Ginger, Spinach Soup

Extra Boost
Papaya, Peach & Pear Crush

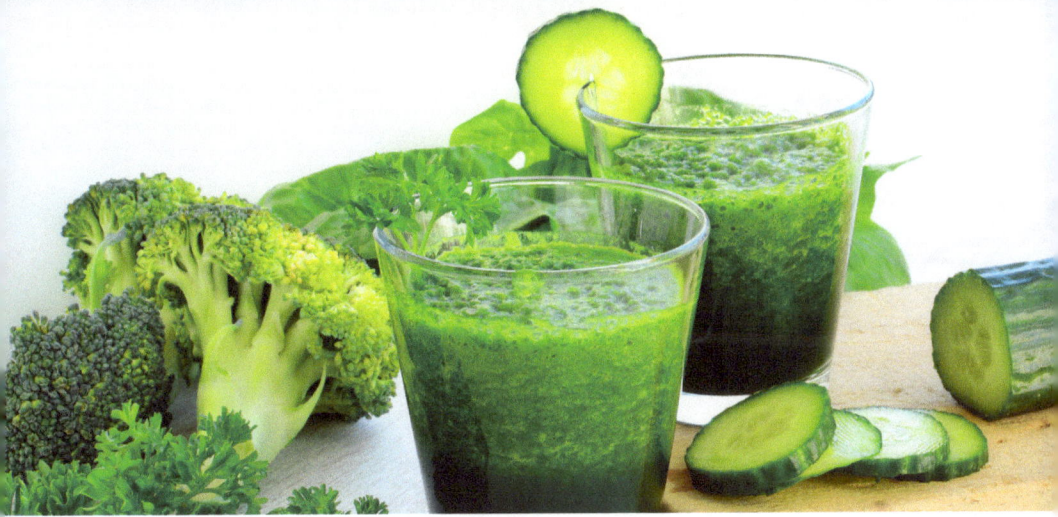

Broccoli Power Juice

3 broccoli stem

½ cucumber

1 asparagus

1 parsnip

1 celery

2 green apples

2 cm root ginger

Wash produce. Core apples. Chop vegetables to size, to fit juicer. Juice all vegetables and fruits in a juicer.

FOOD	NUTRITIONAL BENEFITS
Broccoli	Builds collagen - forms tissue and bone. Antioxidant.
Cucumber	Stress relief, hydration, skin health
Asparagus	Helps fight cancer, good for cleansing blood, richin fibre, diuretic
Parsnip	High in potassium: Reduce blood pressure. Improve heart health.
Celery	Rich in antioxidants and beneficial enzymes
Apples	Cleanse colon, regulate blood sugar, lower cholesterol
Ginger	Powerful anti-inflammatory (good for arthritis), soothes stomach

Spinach Energy Smoothie

Handful spinach

1 avocado

½ pineapple

1 large carrot

½ medium banana

Hemp seed oil

½ lemon unwaxed

375 ml coconut water

Peel banana, avocado and lemon. Dice beetroot, pineapple and carrot. Put all ingredients in a smoothie machine with coconut water and blend. Add spinach and hemp seed oil until smooth.

FOOD	NUTRITIONAL BENEFITS
Spinach	Superfood, nutrient-rich - skin, hair and bone health
Avocado	Fibre-rich, heart healthy, brain healthy, good for the nervous system
Pineapple	Eye health, enzyme rich, reduce allergies, ease digestion
Carrot	Rich in beta-carotene: for healthy skin, immune system & eye health
Banana	Fibre rich, ease digestion, prevent anaemia
Hemp seed oil	Mineral-rich, hormone balancing, great for vegetarians and vegans
Lemon	Anti-parasitic, alkalizing all round cleanser
Coconut water	Hydration. Electrolytes. Antioxidant.

Butternut, Ginger & Spinach Soup

Day 15 soup mixture

Handful spinach

Parsley to garnish

1 stalk mint

Use the rest of day 15 soup. Add spinach, simmer for 5 minutes then add parsley chopped parsley to garnish

FOOD	NUTRITIONAL BENEFITS
Spinach	Super food, nutrient-rich - skin, hair and bone health
Parsley	Good for kidney and bladder health. Cleanses & relieves constipation
Butternut Squash	Good for bones, eyesight, skin and relieves constipation
Ginger	Powerful anti-inflammatory (good for arthritis), soothes the stomach

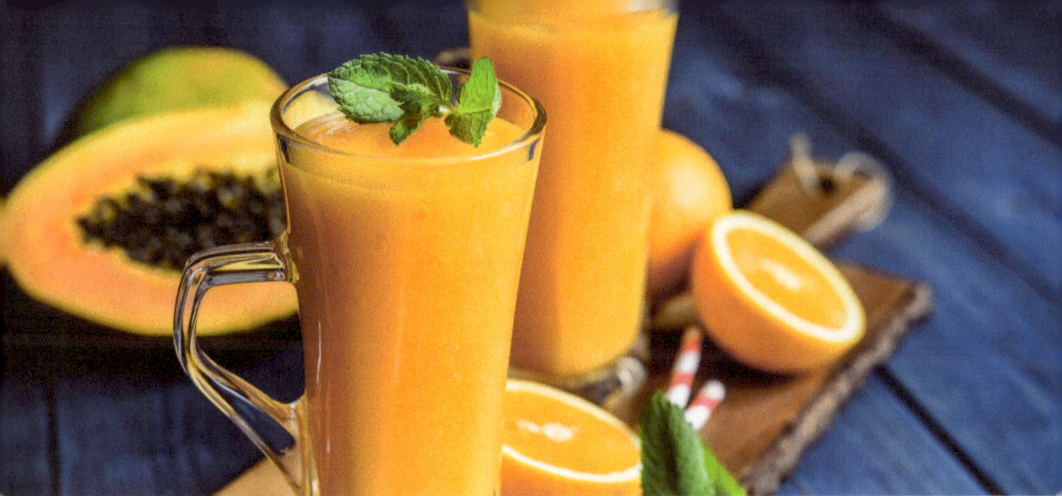

Papaya, Peach & Pear Crush

1 unwaxed lemon

½ papaya

1 peach

1 pear

1 stalk mint

400 ml water

Peel lemon and papaya. Cut lemon, papaya, peach and pear in chunks. Add to a smoothie machine. Blend until smooth, then add mint.

FOOD	NUTRITIONAL BENEFITS
Lemon	Anti-parasitic, alkalizing all round cleanser
Papaya	Eye health, improves digestion, weight loss aid. Anti-diabetic.
Peach	Immune system booster, relief from cancer. Antioxidants. Skin health.
Pear	Calms nerves, supple joints, and good for gout/ arthritis. Mild laxative.
Mint	Aids in digestion. Antiseptic, antibacterial, helps IBS & headaches

DAY 17

Breakfast
Spinach, Mint & Pear Juice

Lunch
Papaya & Mango Smoothie

Dinner
Celery, Spinach & Carrot Soup

Extra Boost
Passion Fruit Chiller

Spinach, Mint & Pear Juice

250 ml coconut water

Handful of spinach

2 pears (chopped)

1 stalk mint

Wash produce. Add spinach and then mint to the juicer first. Then juice the pears.

FOOD	NUTRITIONAL BENEFITS
Spinach	Super food, nutrient-rich - skin, hair and bone health
Pears	Calms nerves, supple joints, and good for gout/arthritis. Mild laxative.
Mint	Aids in digestion. Antiseptic, antibacterial, helps IBS & headaches

Papaya & Mango Smoothie

1 papaya (chopped)   Handful of watercress
1 mango (chopped)   Handful parsley
2 limes   500 ml coconut water

Peel Papaya, mango and lime. Juice all vegetables and fruits in a juicer. Remembering to juice the greens first. Add coconut water to taste.

FOOD	NUTRITIONAL BENEFITS
Papaya	Eye health, improves digestion, weight loss aid. Anti-diabetic.
Mango	Skin and eye health. Helps fight cancer. Improves digestion
Lime	Cleanses blood, improves digestion and great for thyroid health.
Watercress	Protects against cancer, antioxidant, bone & teeth strength.
Parsley	Good for kidney and bladder health. Cleanses & relieves constipation
Coconut Water	Hydration. Electrolytes. Antioxidant.

Spinach, Celery & Carrot Soup

2 carrots (chopped)

1 celery

1 leek

Handful spinach

Coriander

Himalayan salt

1 litre water

Wash produce. Dice carrots and celery. Add carrots, celery and leek to boiling water. Boiled for 20 minutes. Add coriander and salt to taste.

Optional: leave to cool. Add mixture to smoothie machine, blend until smooth.

FOOD	NUTRITIONAL BENEFITS
Carrot	Rich in beta-carotene: for healthy skin, immune system & eye health
Celery	Rich in antioxidants and beneficial enzymes
Leek	Fight free radicals in your body. Anti-cancer. Anti-diabetes.
Spinach	Super food, nutrient-rich - skin, hair and bone health
Coriander	Cleansing, reduce infections, lower blood sugars
Himalayan salt	Balance pH and blood sugar. Detoxify body. Improves hydration.

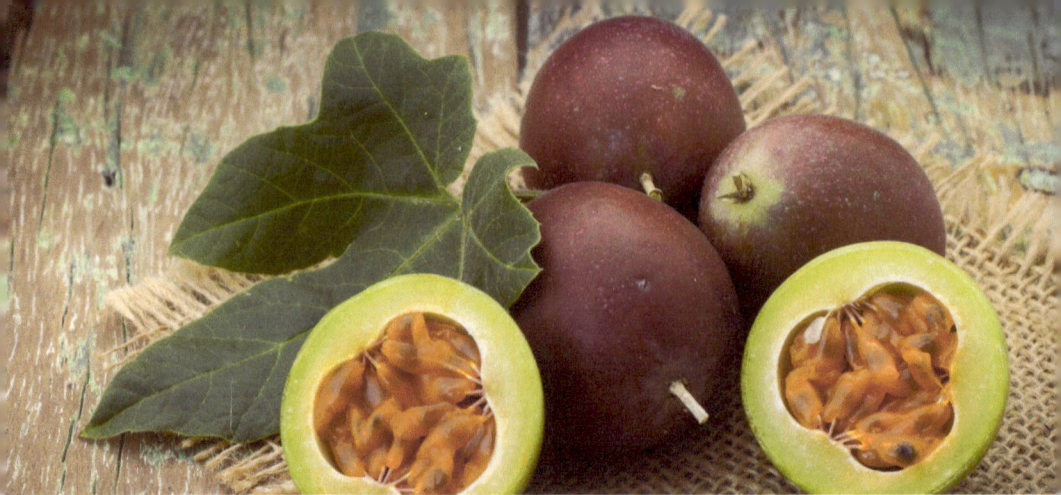

Passion Fruit Chiller

2 passion fruits	1 unwaxed lime
1 stalk mint	375 ml water
1 apple	

Peel and remove seeds from passion fruit. Peel lemon. Core apple. Juice unwaxed lime and apple in a juicer. Add juice to a smoothie machine with passion fruit. Blend until smooth, then add mint.

FOOD	NUTRITIONAL BENEFITS
Lime	Cleanses blood, improves digestion and great for thyroid health.
Passion fruit	Immune system booster, aids digestion, anti-cancer, improves circulation
Mint	Aids in digestion. Antiseptic, antibacterial, helps IBS & headaches
Apple	Cleanse colon, regulate blood sugar, lower cholesterol

DAY 18

Breakfast
Grapefruit & Orange Juice

Lunch
Kale, Fennel & Lime Delight

Dinner
Coconut & Sweet Potato Soup

Extra Boost
Cherry & Strawberry Blast

Grapefruit & Orange Juice

1 grapefruit

1 large orange (chopped)

1 stalk parsley

Peel grapefruit and orange. Juice grapefruit, parsley and orange in a juicer.

FOOD	NUTRITIONAL BENEFITS
Grapefruit	Maintain a healthy heart and blood pressure
Orange	Anti-diabetes, skin food, heart healthy, anti-cancer, vitamin c rich
Parsley	Good for kidney and bladder health. Cleanses & relieves constipation

Kale, Fennel & Lime Delight

Handful of kale

1 fennel (chopped)

1 lime

1 golden delicious apple

Pumpkin seed

Avocado oil

Wash produce. Peel lime. Core apple. Place chopped apple, fennel, kale and lime to a juicer. Add pumpkin seed and a drizzle of avocado oil.

FOOD	NUTRITIONAL BENEFITS
Kale	High in iron, zero fat, prevent cancer, anti-inflammatory
Fennel	Cleansing benefits, rich in vitamin B6, antioxidant rich, calcium rich
Lime	Cleanses blood, improves digestion and great for thyroid health.
Apple	Cleanse colon, regulate blood sugar, lower cholesterol
Pumpkin seed	Nutritional powerhouse, good for nerves, antioxidant, protein rich
Avocado oil	Heart healthy, brain healthy, good for nervous system

Coconut & Sweet Potato Soup

1 leek

1 celery stalk

100 ml coconut cream

1 small sweet potato

1 large carrot

Coriander

Himalayan salt

1 litre water

Peel and chop sweet potato. Add coconut cream and sweet potato to leek, celery, and carrots. Bring to boil for 10 minutes. Add coriander and salt to taste.

FOOD	NUTRITIONAL BENEFITS
Coconut cream	Lowers Blood Pressure & Cholesterol. Helps Prevent Anaemia
Sweet potato	Super food. Good for diabetes. Anti-cancer. Immune system booster.
Coriander	Cleansing, reduce infections, lower blood sugars
Himalayan salt	Balance pH and blood sugar. Detoxify body. Improves hydration
Carrot	Rich in beta-carotene: for healthy skin, immune system & eye health
Celery	Rich in antioxidants and beneficial enzymes
Leek	Fight free radicals in your body. Anti-cancer and anti-diabetes.

Cherry & Strawberry Blast

1 unwaxed lemon

Handful strawberries

1 stalk mint

15 cherries (chopped)

300 ml water

Juice unwaxed lemon in a juicer. Add juice to a smoothie machine with cherries and strawberries. Blend until smooth, then add mint.

FOOD	NUTRITIONAL BENEFITS
Cherries	Reduce belly fat, promote healthy sleep, antioxidant-rich, reduce muscle pain
Lemon	Anti-parasitic, alkalizing all round cleanser
Strawberries	Overall health, rich in vitamins, fibre and minerals.
Mint	Aids in digestion. Antiseptic, antibacterial, helps IBS & headaches

DAY 19

Breakfast
Pineapple, Cucumber & Red Cabbage Juice

Lunch
Tomato Smoothie

Dinner
Pea and Pumpkin Soup

Extra Boost
Broccoli and Lime Blast

Pineapple, Cucumber & Red Cabbage Juice

½ cucumber

½ pineapple (chopped)

1 unwaxed lime

1 celery

1 Apple

Handful of kale

Handful of watercress

¼ red cabbage

Handful spinach

Juice cucumber, pineapple, lime, celery, kale, watercress, cabbage and spinach in a juicer.

FOOD	NUTRITIONAL BENEFITS
Cucumber	Stress relief, hydration, skin health
Pineapple	Eye health, enzyme rich, reduce allergies, ease digestion
Lime	Cleanses blood, improves digestion and great for thyroid health.
Celery	Rich in antioxidants and beneficial enzymes
Kale	High in iron, zero fat, prevent cancer, anti-inflammatory
Watercress	Protects against cancer, antioxidant, bone & teeth strength. Anti-parasitic, alkalizing all round cleanser
Red Cabbage	Prevents aging, diabetes, strengthens immune system, helps weight loss. Improves skin, eye, stronger bones, eliminates toxic substances
Spinach	Super food, nutrient rich - skin, hair and bone health

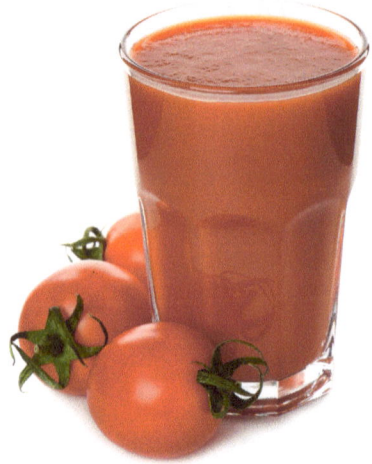

Tomato Smoothie

1 large tomato

1 avocado

1 unwaxed lemon

1 cm red chili

500 ml water

Wash produce. Peel lemon and avocado (removing seed). Cut end of chili and chop tomatoes. Place chopped tomato, avocado, lemon and chili in a smoothie machine with water. Blend until smooth.

FOOD	NUTRITIONAL BENEFITS
Tomato	Antioxidant, anti-cancer, eye health, digestive comfort, manage diabetes
Avocado	Fiber rich, heart healthy, brain healthy, good for nervous system
Lemon	Anti-parasitic, alkalizing all round cleanser
Chili	Cleanse sinus, aids digestion, relieve migraine & muscle pain

Pea & Pumpkin Soup

1 onion

1 small packet green peas

1 celery stalk

1 leek

¼ pumpkin

1 sweet potato

Parsley

Thyme

Himalayan salt

Peel and dice onion. Peel and chop sweet potato into cubes. Add pumpkin, celery, onion, and sweet potato, bring to boil for 20 minutes. Add thyme, coriander and salt, cook for a further 3 minutes.

FOOD	NUTRITIONAL BENEFITS
Pumpkin	Soothe digestive tract, boost vision, healthy heart
Celery	Rich in antioxidants and beneficial enzymes
Leek	Fight free radicals in your body. Anti-cancer. Anti-diabetes.
Onion	Balance blood sugar. Cancer-fighting.
Sweet potato	Superfood. Good for diabetes. Anti-cancer. Immune system booster.
Parsley	Good for kidney and bladder health. Cleanses & relieves constipation
Thyme	Healing properties, good for digestion, diuretic.
Himalayan salt	Balance pH and blood sugar. Detoxify body. Improves hydration.
Green Peas	Good source of dietary fibre, Vitamin A, iron, folate, thiamin, Vitamin C, K and manganese. Helps to control blood sugar.

Broccoli and Lime Blast

125 ml water

3 stem broccoli

1 unwaxed lime

Handful of spinach

Peel lime. Juice unwaxed lemon in a juicer. Add juice to a smoothie machine with broccoli and spinach. Blend until smooth.

FOOD	NUTRITIONAL BENEFITS
Broccoli	Builds collagen - forms tissue and bone. Antioxidant.
Lime	Cleanses blood, improves digestion and great for thyroid health.
Spinach	Super food, nutrient rich - skin, hair and bone health

DAY 20

Breakfast
Asparagus, broccoli & Celery Juice

Lunch
Carrot & Ginger Drink

Dinner
Minestrone Soup

Extra Boost
Plum Chiller

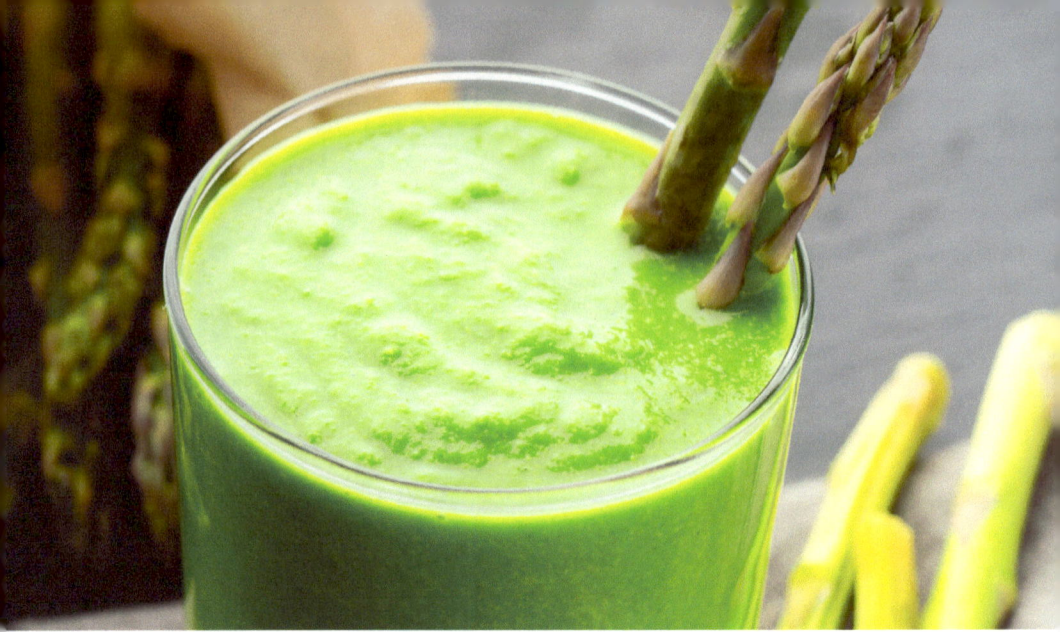

Asparagus, Broccoli and Celery Juice

3 stalks asparagus

½ cucumber

3 stems broccoli

2 cm ginger

2 green apples

1 celery

1 parsnip

Handful spinach

Wash produce. Core apples. Cut produce to size. Juice cucumber, asparagus, broccoli, ginger, celery, parsnip, apples and spinach in a juicer.

FOOD	NUTRITIONAL BENEFITS
Asparagus	Helps fight cancer, good for cleansing blood, rich in fibre, diuretic
Cucumber	Stress relief, hydration, skin health
Broccoli	Builds collagen - forms tissue and bone. Antioxidant.
Ginger	Powerful anti-inflammatory (good for arthritis), soothes the stomach
Apples	Cleanse colon, regulate blood sugar, lower cholesterol
Celery	Rich in antioxidants and beneficial enzymes
Parsnip	High in potassium: Reduce blood pressure. Improve heart health.
Spinach	Superfood, nutrient-rich - skin, hair and bone health

Carrot & Ginger Drink

3 large carrots   ½ cucumber

3 cm ginger   2 cm red chili

Handful watercress

Wash produce. Cut to size. Place chopped carrots, ginger, cucumber, chili and watercress in the juicer.

FOOD	NUTRITIONAL BENEFITS
Carrots	Rich in beta-carotene: for healthy skin, immune system & eye health
Ginger	Powerful anti-inflammatory (good for arthritis), soothes the stomach
Watercress	Protects against cancer, antioxidant, bone & teeth strength.
Cucumber	Stress relief, hydration, skin health
Chilli	Cleanse sinus, aids digestion, relieve migraine & muscle pain

Minestrone Soup

1 onion (chopped)

3 celery (chopped)

2 cloves garlic

¼ green cabbage (chopped)

Himalayan salt

Handful of green peas

1 large tomato (chopped)

Coriander

Thyme

Wash produce. Peel and crush/ finely chop garlic. Peel and dice onion. Add onion, celery, garlic, cabbage and peas bring to boil for 20 minutes. Add thyme, coriander, tomato and salt, cook for a further 3 minutes.

FOOD	NUTRITIONAL BENEFITS
Onion	Balance blood sugar. Cancer fighting.
Celery	Rich in antioxidants and beneficial enzymes
Garlic	Neutralize free radicals preventing cellular damage.
Green cabbage	Fights inflammation, promotes healthy gut, combats chronic disease
Olive oil	Antioxidant rich, anti-inflammatory, prevent strokes, heart healthy
Tomato	Antioxidant, anti-cancer, eye health, digestive comfort, manage diabetes
Thyme	Healing properties, good for digestion, diuretic.
Coriander	Cleansing, reduce infections, lower blood sugars
Himalayan salt	Balance pH and blood sugar. Detoxify body. Improves hydration.

Plum Chiller

3 plums

1 unwaxed lemon

200 ml coconut water

1 stalk mint

Juice unwaxed lemon in a juicer. Remove stone from plums. Add juice to a smoothie machine with plums and coconut water. Blend until smooth.

FOOD	NUTRITIONAL BENEFITS
Plums	Vitamin C rich, great for constipation/ IBS.
Lemon	Anti-parasitic, alkalizing all round cleanser
Coconut Water	Hydration. Electrolytes. Antioxidant.
Mint	Aids in digestion. Antiseptic, antibacterial, helps IBS & headaches

DAY 21

Hallelujah!!!!

Well done for keeping up with your juice, smoothie and soup fast.
You must feel & look amazing and energized!!!!

Breakfast
Banana, Berries & Nut Smoothie

Lunch
Ginger & Grapefruit Juice

Dinner
Coconut, Butternut Squash & Carrot Soup

Extra Boost
Peach Chiller

Banana, Berries & Nut Smoothie

Mixed seeds (pumpkin, sunflower)   1 ripe banana

375 ml coconut water   15 almonds

Berries (strawberry, raspberries, blueberries)

Peel banana. Pour coconut water in the smoothie machine. Add berries, banana, almonds and mixed seeds. Blend until smoothie.

FOOD	NUTRITIONAL BENEFITS
Pumpkin seeds	A nutritional powerhouse, good for nerves, anti-oxidant, protein-rich
Sunflower Seeds	Heart-healthy, antioxidant, good for thyroid health and mood.
Almonds	Relieves Stress. May prevent cardiovascular disease.
Banana	Fibre rich, ease digestion, prevent anaemia
Berries	Overall health, rich in vitamins, fiber, minerals.
Coconut water	Hydration. Electrolytes. Antioxidant.

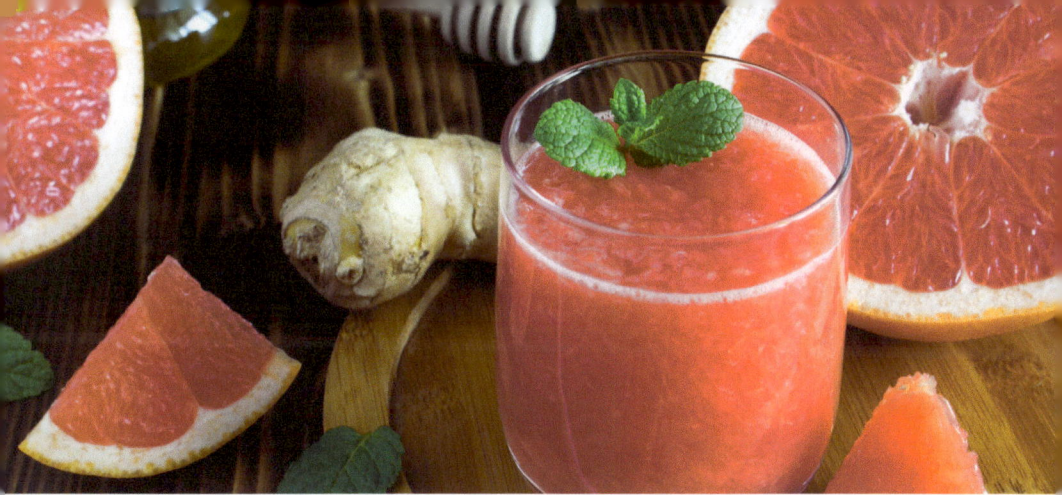

Ginger & Grapefruit Juice

1 grapefruit

3 cm ginger

1 unwaxed lime

1 apple (golden delicious)

¼ pineapple

Hemp oil

Wash produce. Core apple. Peel grapefruit and lime. Peel and dice pineapple. Place chopped grapefruit, ginger, apple, lime and pineapple in the juicer.

FOOD	NUTRITIONAL BENEFITS
Grapefruit	Maintain a healthy heart and blood pressure
Ginger	Powerful anti-inflammatory (good for arthritis), soothes the stomach
Lime	Cleanses blood, improves digestion and great for thyroid health.
Apple	Cleanse colon, regulate blood sugar, lower cholesterol
Pineapple	Eye health, enzyme rich, reduce allergies, ease digestion
Hemp oil	Mineral-rich, hormone balancing, great for vegetarians and vegans

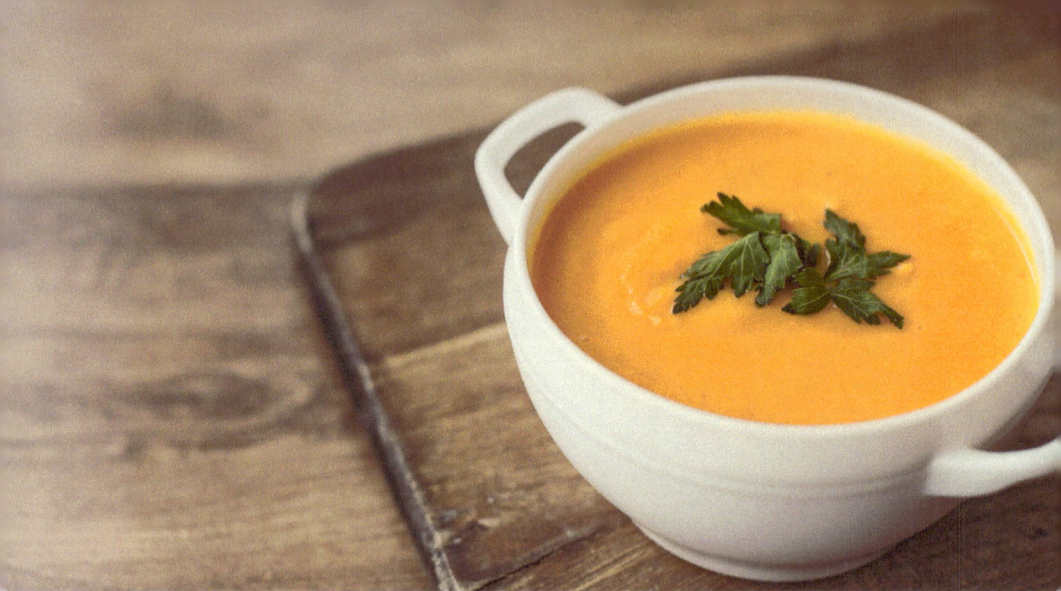

Coconut, Butternut Squash & Carrot Soup

1 onion (chopped)

¼ butternut squash (chopped)

2 cloves garlic

200 ml coconut milk

2 large carrots (chopped)

Parsley

3 cm chili pepper

Himalayan salt

Peel and chop onion. Peel and dice butternut squash. Crush or finely chop garlic. Wash and chop carrots and parsley. Add onion, butternut squash, garlic, carrots and parsley with coconut water, bring to boil for 20 minutes. Add chili pepper, parsley and salt, cook for a further 3 minutes. Leave to cool, then transfer to a smoothie machine and blend until smooth.

FOOD	NUTRITIONAL BENEFITS
Onion	Balance blood sugar. Cancer-fighting.
Butternut squash	Good for bones, eyesight, skin and relieves constipation
Garlic	Neutralize free radicals preventing cellular damage.
Coconut milk	Lowers Blood Pressure & Cholesterol. Helps Prevent Anaemia
Carrots	Rich in beta-carotene: for healthy skin, immune system & eye health
Parsley	Good for kidney and bladder health. Cleanses & relieves constipation
Chilli	Cleanse sinus, aids digestion, relieve migraine & muscle pain

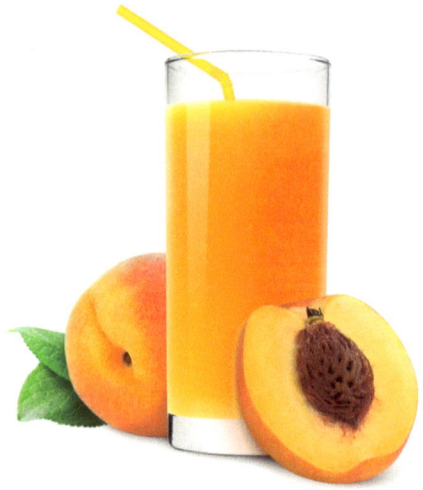

Peach Chiller

2 peach (chopped)

1 apple

1 unwaxed lime

250 ml coconut water

1 stalk parsley

Juice unwaxed lime in a juicer. Core apple. Peel lime. Remove stone from peach. Add juice to a smoothie machine with peach, apple, parsley and coconut water. Blend until smooth.

FOOD	NUTRITIONAL BENEFITS
Peach	Immune system booster, relief from cancer. Antioxidants. Skin health.
Apple	Cleanse colon, regulate blood sugar, lower cholesterol
Lime	Cleanses blood, improves digestion and great for thyroid health.
Coconut water	Hydration. Electrolytes. Antioxidant.
Parsley	Good for kidney and bladder health. Cleanses & relieves constipation

Glossary

Acrylamide: A chemical that forms in some foods during high-temperature cooking processes and is a known neurotoxin.

Activated Charcoal: Also known as activated carbon, used to trap toxins and chemicals in the body, allowing them to be flushed out so the body doesn't reabsorb them.

Amino Acid: The building blocks of Protein, crucial to almost all biological processes.

Antibacterial Anything that destroys bacteria or suppresses their growth or their ability to reproduce. Normally, when we are talking about reducing bacteria in our health, we are talking about "bad" bacteria that can cause infection

Anti-fungal: Something that limits or prevents the growth of yeasts and other fungal organisms.

Anti-inflammatory: Substance that reduces inflammation or swelling

Antioxidant: Removes damaging oxidizing agents in a living organism.

Anti-Parasitic: Something that limits or prevents the growth of parasites.

Artificial Food Dye: Synthetic food dyes (or colourings) that do not exist in nature. Some of which are detrimental to our health.

Bacteria: Good and Bad bacteria are simple organisms that live everywhere in the earth. "Good" Bacteria is bacteria thought to be beneficial for our health. "Bad" bacteria, is bacteria that is not beneficial to our health

Beta carotene: Beta-Carotene helps our body create Vitamin A. Found in bright orange compounds. Great for our mucous membranes and skin health.

Carcinogenesis: The initiation of cancer formation.

Carcinogens: A substance that can cause cancer in living tissue.

Castor Oil: A vegetable oil obtained by pressing the seeds of the castor oil plant. Beneficial for skin, hair and overall health.

Cellular damage: When a cell is adversely affected by a chemical, infectious, biological or nutritional factor. It can be reversible or irreversible.

Cholesterol: An organic lipid molecule vital for the normal functioning of the body. Made by the liver, but can also be found in some foods.

Chronic disease: A human health condition or disease that comes with time. Is persistent or otherwise long-lasting in its effects.

Developmental Toxins: A toxin that causes a structural or functional alteration, that interferes with homeostasis, normal growth, differentiation, development or behaviour, and which is caused by environment or lifestyle.

Electrolytes: A substance that produces an electrically conducting solution when dissolved water or solvent.

Endocrine system: A collection of glands that produce hormones that regulate just about every function in the body.

Enzymes: Used for most biochemical reactions in living things. Enzymes are protein molecules in cells which work as catalysts that speed up chemical reactions in the body.

Epsom Salts: Made of magnesium sulphate. A pure, time-tested mineral compound with many uses, from creating at-home spas to soothing achy muscles.

EWG: Environmental Working Group

Fasting: The willing abstinence or reduction from some or all food, drink, or both, for a period

Free radicals: Very dangerous for our health. Can start a chain reaction, like dominoes. React with important cellular components such as DNA, or the cell membrane. Making cells perform poorly or die if this occurs.

Fungus: Microorganisms also are known as: Fungi, fungi. Fungus, plural fungi, any of about 99,000 known species of organisms of the kingdom Fungi, which includes the yeasts, rusts, smuts, mildews, molds, and mushrooms.

Good fats: Both mono- and polyunsaturated fats, can help lower cholesterol levels and reduce your risk of heart disease.

Gut flora: AKA. Gut microbiota or gastrointestinal microbiota is the complex community of microorganisms that live in the digestive tracts of humans and other animals, including insects

Herbicides: Control specific weed species, while leaving crops unharmed. However can be harmful to our health.

HFCS: High fructose corn syrup

Hormone disruptors: Chemicals that can interfere with endocrine (or hormone) systems (see endocrine system above)

IBS: Irritable bowel syndrome, is a long-term disease of the digestive system. It can cause bouts of stomach cramps, bloating, diarrhoea and constipation.

Immune system: The body's defense against infectious organisms and other invaders.

Irradiation: The process by which an object is exposed to radiation. The process produces a similar effect to pasteurisation in our food.

Magnesium: Magnesium supplements are a great idea, as 80% of the population are magnesium deficient. Magnesium plays a large role in a lot of the bodies vital systems.

MSG: Monosodium glutamate is a naturally occurring non-essential amino acid. Used as a flavour enhancer, linked to various health problems, such as headaches and allergic reactions.

Mutagenesis: A process by which the genetic information of an organism is changed, resulting in a mutation

Neurotoxins: Toxins that are poisonous or destructive to nerve tissue

Parasites: Can live on or in a host and feed off of it.

Pesticides: Chemical compounds used to kill pests, including insects, rodents, fungi and weeds.

Phytochemicals: Chemical compounds produced by plants, generally to help them thrive or ward off competitors, predators, or pathogens

SAD: Standard American Diet, consumed worldwide - rich in red meat, dairy products, processed and artificially sweetened foods, and salt, with minimal intake of fruits, vegetables, fish, legumes, and whole grains.

Index

O

Organic foods, 11
Oxygenated aldehydes, 15

P

Parasites, 11, 154, 157
Pesticides, 11-12, 24, 157
Phytochemicals 15, 69, 157
Preservatives, 25

R

Reproductive dysfunction, 11
Reproductive toxins, 11

S

Standard American Diet (SAD),
14, 157

T

Toxicity, 11
Toxins, 10-11, 27, 154, 155, 157

V

Vitamins, 6, 16, 20, 51, 79, 112, 135,
148

W

Weight loss, 16, 42, 51, 125, 128
World Health Organization, 11

Y

Yeast, 11, 154, 156

Recipe Index

10% OFF
when you buy

BODY BALANCE JUICE PROGRAMME – DETOX JOURNAL

Thank you for sharing this journey with me!

www.ingramcontent.com/pod-product-compliance
Lightning Source LLC
Chambersburg PA
CBHW040126270326
41926CB00005B/87